# Becoming Doctors

## The Adoption of a Cloak of Competence

**A VOLUME IN**
**CONTEMPORARY ETHNOGRAPHIC STUDIES**

*Editor:* Jaber F. Gubrium, *Department of Sociology, University of Florida*

# CONTEMPORARY ETHNOGRAPHIC STUDIES

Editor: **Jaber F. Gubrium**
*Department of Sociology*
*University of Florida*

*To my mother, Harriet Haas,*
*for her courage and example*
*Jack Haas*


*To my wife and children*
*parents and sister*
*William Shaffir*

# Becoming Doctors

## The Adoption of a Cloak of Competence

**Jack Haas**
**William Shaffir**
*Department of Sociology*
*McMaster University*

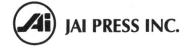 **JAI PRESS INC.**

*Greenwich, Connecticut*                    *London, England*

**Library of Congress Cataloging-in-Publication Data**

Haas, Jack, 1939—
   Becoming doctors.

   (Contemporary ethnographic studies)
   Bibliography: p.
   Includes index.
   1. Medical colleges—Canada—Sociological aspects.
2. Medical students—Canada—Social conditions.
3. Medical students—Canada—Attitudes. 4. Professional
socialization—Canada. I. Shaffir, William. II. Title.
III. Series [DNLM: 1. Attitude of Health Personnel.
2. Clinical Competence. 3. Education, Medical.
4. Students, Medical. W  18  H112b]
R749.H23   1987   610'.7'1171   87-2858
ISBN 1-55938-408-5

# Contents

# *Preface*

*Becoming Doctors: The Adoption of Cloak of Competence* is an intimate portrayal of medical school socialization in an innovative medical school. Through first hand participant observation and informal interviews we describe student perceptions and adaptations to the process. This begins at admissions and ends at graduation. Comparisons and contrasts with those of students in more traditional professional programs are noted. The result is an attempt to integrate and synthesize these findings into an holistic conception of professionalization.

The emphasis throughout has been on generating and testing hypotheses and concepts, thus producing an analytic model which describes the true nature of professionalization. The comparative method has aided this effort and helped to unveil the shrouds of mystification and ideology that characterize this process at the individual, group, organizational and occupational levels. We have found that the exaggerated expectations and claims that surround the profession and the professional role require exaggerated adaptations and efforts of legitimation.

Although our interest was not evaluative and the locus of study is incidental to our conclusions, the medical school we studied is, necessarily, critically examined. If our interest had been evaluative, we would also have reported some very positive aspects of the program and the fact that students were generally enthusiastic about McMaster and its innovative curricula. It is also important for us to note that our interest in this socialization process essentially ignores the curriculum context and student acquisition of medical knowledge and skills. Our interest as sociologists gives emphasis to the art, rather than the science of medicine and to the "hidden curriculum" of professionalization. We regret any perceived imbalance by some of the school's administrators, but maintain that our findings are not specific to the school we studied. In effect, they reveal and illustrate the more general characteristics of professionalization. We have been encouraged about the validity of our analysis by the students we studied. These students provided continuous feedback about our analysis, as did our professional colleagues and peers who have read and commented favorably about our work.

This book is the culmination of a long and sometimes difficult research process. When the idea first emerged to do a "Boys in White" study of an innovative school, we never fully grasped the time, energy, strains and commitment such an enterprise would involve. Now as the process is completed, we can retrospectively appreciate the difficult times. One enduring highlight is the comfortable and secure relationship that developed between the co-authors. In the sometimes petty and competitive world of professional life, it is often difficult for people to cooperate, let alone enjoy their work together. Our relationship gives testimony to the idea that joint research and writing can be a joy if the individuals take the work and the relationship more seriously than themselves.

Our largest debt of gratitude is to the students of this study whose generous cooperation and interest made the study possible. Their support opened many doors that might otherwise have been closed. We are grateful to the faculty and practitioners at the medical school who facilitated our research and allowed us into their tutorials and clinical settings.

# Acknowledgments

The author's of *Becoming Doctors: The Adoption of a Cloak of Competence,* wish to thank the Canada Council and McMaster University for grants that supported the research and paid for the very large typwriting costs. We especially want to thank Dean Peter George for providing us with funds at critical times. Ms. Lee d'Anjou and Mrs. Barbara Brown provided very helpful editorial advice and insights at various stages. Professor Victor M. Marshall currently affiliated with the Department of Behavioural Sciences, University of Toronto, participated in this study for the first year and a half. He was involved in the data collection phase and helped shape the analysis during this period. We would also like to express our gratitude to the secretaries of the Department of Sociology, particularly Mrs. Shirley McGill, Ms. Chris Downey and Ms. Jackie Tucker for their prompt servicing of our typing needs.

In closing we would like to thank the following for their helpful comments and suggestions: Howard S. Becker, Leo Cellini, C.E. Berkeley Fleming, Ronald Keyser, Sherryl Kleinman, Victor M. Marshall, Robert Prus, Malcolm Spector, and Roger Thomas. We accept, however, full responsibility for the final product. We would like to acknowledge the following permissions.

Haas, Jack, and William Shaffir, "The Fate of Idealism Revisited," *Urban Life,* vol. 13, no. 1, pp. 63–81. Copyright © 1984 by Sage Publications. Reprinted with permission.

From Fieldwork Experience: Qualitative Approaches to Social Research by William B. Shaffir, Robert A. Stebbins, and Allan Turowetz. Copyright © 1980 by St. Martin's Press, Inc., and used with permission.

# Chapter I

# *Towards a Theory of Professionalization*

In this book, we attempt to analyze the professionalization of medical students. Our study (based on participant observation) was carried out within the context of a medical school with an extremely innovative curriculum.[1] Although primarily concerned with this particular program, the study extended its scope to include comparisons with the programs of more traditional medical schools. In both types of schools, we note the centrality of the concept of legitimation. The effective control and manipulation of people, ideas, and symbols, provides aspiring and practicing medical professionals with the means by which they can control the definition of the situation—that of "professed" authority. While we did not concern ourselves in any detailed way with professions other than medicine, the model we develop in this work can be profitably applied to the professionalization process in other occupations that demand its workers project an image of trustworthy competence to their clients.

Reviewing the research about the nature of the professions added to a synthesis of our own observations. In addition, analysis of medical student socialization has allowed us to reach certain conclusions about the process of professionalization. By contrasting the process by which an occupation makes and is accorded its claim to professional status, we note the similarities with the professionalization of its members. Before examining the nature of student socialization into a profession, we will

1

examine the analogous process of occupational profession-alization.[2]

In order for an occupation to achieve professional status, it must be granted legitimacy by whatever audience that is crucial to such status passage. That audience may include clients, "public", or the state. A profession is by definition a social object that has effectively convinced these important others that the socially accepted characteristics it claims or "professes" are valid (Ritzer, 1977; Wilensky, 1964; Montagna, 1977). The occupation symbolizes (Becker, 1962) the appropriate at-tributes, skills, and/or knowledge creating a distinctive identity that is the basis for its legitimate authority over certain moral issues. Through the manipulation of symbols, ideas and peo-ple, the occupational group seeks, and is eventually accorded, a legitimated monopoly. In turn this formal or licensed status makes the claim official and bureaucratic. The occupation is granted the "license and mandate" (Hughes, 1959) to intercede in the important human matters of disease and death, liberty and property, and good and evil (Goode, 1957).

Indeterminancy and uncertainty in these weighty matters is believed to be ameliorated by the intervention of those "chosen" or qualified by their convincing demonstrations of "special" attributes, skills and/or knowledge (characteristics of charisma) (Etzioni, 1975). These attributes become routinized and invested in the office or social status of the professional. The charismatic or quasi-religious nature of the role is rooted in the moral nature of the professional enterprise. The elusive nature of this morality is characterized by uncertainty, indeter-minancy, and an absence of routine. This is necessarily accom-plished only by those who themselves symbolize, through pro-cess of mystification, a special or transcendental authority.

In primitive societies, the monopoly over the irrational mat-ters of human life was typically embodied in charistmatic indi-viduals. It was the medicine man or the shaman, as he was called, who was first considered to have the ability to interface with the spirit world. He was believed to have the power to give the dead safe rites of passage to the afterlife. An extension of this role empowered him with the ability to influence those spirits concerned with the dissemination of disease. Thus the shaman assumed the triple role of priest, sorcerer and physician, addressing the human need of man to triumph over death and evil (Becker, 1975).

Increasingly, this overt manipulation of others through religious symbols and ideas was replaced by those rooted in principles and findings of science. Scientific knowledge grew, accompanied by the increasing secularization of society, creating a new basis for intervention in those areas of human concern, once the province of the shaman, was developed. The Industrial Revolution fed into this "forward" march and the more universalistic principles of science gained strength as the core characteristic of demonstrated competence and superior expertise (Larson, 1977). The secular basis of professionalism was, however, maintained as the exclusive preserve of those who had access to the mysteries of science. The mystification was exacerbated through the use of esoteric language in law, medicine and religion, combined with the less overt vestiges of sacred symbols and rituals, consequently reinforcing the special and privileged status of those specially prepared to participate in ritual ordeals. Professional authority thus remains rooted in sacred-power which represents immortality power (Becker, 1975:49). The law, though still rooted more in moral matters than scientific principles, relies on ritual enactments of justice as the sacred basis of authority (Wilensky, 1964).

In the prescientific period, medicine was the domain of religion and the art of modern medicine still remains rooted in mystery and ritual. All doctrines which focus on the good of humanity have religious symbolism as a basis (Collins, 1982) and medicine has been effectively analyzed as a state religion (Freidson, 1970; Mendelson, 1979) with physicians serving as the new priests of secular society.

In sum, the basis of the traditional professions of law, medicine and religion are deeply rooted in religious symbolism which implicitly involves the manipulation of legitimating audiences with symbols and ideas communicating authoritive control in moral matters. These occupations depend on the successful control of legitimators through the use of moral symbols which evoke a taken-for-granted notion of their professed authority. As we will describe, the neophyte learns that the hidden curriculum (Apple, 1971) of professionalization includes a similar requirement. It is to this part of the analysis that our conceptualization of professionalization depends. Professionalization, both of an occupational and individual nature, is rooted in symbolic-ideological legitimation, control and identification.

Professionalization is a process where the "chosen," (those prepared, selected and carefully) convince society, through what is actually the enactment of a moral drama of the myth of their specialness, of their legitimacy to profess and to claim an honorific status (Becker, 1962; Hughes, 1965). The basis of professional dominance centers upon a process by which they mystify their competence. Thus they obscure the basis of their authority, providing the ideological justification for unequal status, closure of access, manipulation of knowledge and control over definitions of the situation (Larson, 1977).

The process of professional socialization or neophyte professionalization thus involves the moral and symbolic transformation of a lay person into the honorific status "professed" by the professional—a process that Davis (1968: 235–251) labels "doctrinal conversion." The neophyte conversion drama involves a liminal process (Turner, 1970) where newcomers face a ritual ordeal (Lortie, 1968; Haas and Shaffir, 1982) as part of this transformation into a sacred identity. The ritual ordeal involved in the process of professionalization is both time-honored and universal. Additionally it demonstrates that only through processes of initiation, analogous to the status passage and development of other master statuses, that society can effectively legitimate the transformation of some members into new moral categories.

In a modern industrial society, the professional school, as part of a scientifically based university, becomes the critical legitimating institution for developing the rites de passage. These rites take the form of what can only be called a dramatic performance or ritual ordeal. The university's scientific basis of authority is the critical symbol system legitimating the monopoly and control over the production of professionals and the selective distribution of professional knowledge and certification (Larson, 1977).

Professionalization can be fruitfully analyzed as a progression in which the neophyte is forced to give a convincing and correct performance in a role that has a specific honorific status. Rigorous processes of selection and preparation, initiation, testing, and threats of humiliation help sustain the myth that the aspirant is undergoing important changes (Kamens, 1977), thus achieving special knowledge, skills, and attributes. The same processes also give the aspirant considerable practice in communicating competence which increases the sense of their trustworthiness. Symbolic changes in wardrobe or costume, props, script, and demeanor both affirm the new role and identity and help to sustain it. Audiences legitimate this performance and thus help to shape an emerging professional identity and a changing conception of the self. In brief, the ritual affects both spectators and participants. The newcomer, through a process of impersonation is accorded, and takes on, a new persona.

A process of ritual ordeal symbolically and psychologically alters professional neophytes. A profession, through its control of the socialization process, also provides newcomers with the justifications for changing their values. The dramatic nature of the conversion process (see Davis, 1968) produces in participants' and spectators' minds the idea that the manipulation and use of symbols and ideas—the control of constructions of reality—is accompanied by, and reflects, appropriate psychological distancing and control.

Professionalization thus involves ritual performances wherein newcomers learn to "play" the professional role, projecting the idea of control and impersonality. The careful staging of these performances protects both clients and professionals alike from identifying with each other, thus preventing any undesirable intrusion of an empathetic response. If the projection of the external professional image is convincing, audiences are induced to exhibit a corresponding control of emotion. Audience and professional collaborate in expecting and producing a certain secularized relationship.

Professionals' interests in monopoly, control, and autonomy are served by the projection of the idea that they are specially trustworthy. The client and other audiences are forced to rely on staged and ritual performances as indicative of an inner psychological control. The ritual dramas that convey a taken-for-granted perspective about trust and special competence move the professional and profession into a new moral category. This category is distanced from lay society and would seem to transcend normal human frailties and limitations. In other words, ritual drama and practices elevate, alienate and separate both profession and professional from society because of "professed" differences. Professionalization can thus be understood as a process of differentiation and alienation from lay society and of the elevation of the professional to a position of detachment and control. Professional relationships typically require professionals to adopt a symbolic-ideological mantle that justifies their special authority in moral matters. Because the role is a moral one, it requires a drama in which players construct convincing performances of their special role.

The essence of professionalization thus involves a process whereby within the structure of the occupation both professional and newcomer convince legitimating audiences about their appropriate competence and trustworthiness in morally fateful matters. Such attributes are communicated by the manipulation and control of symbols, ideas and people. The monopoly and control of legitimating audiences is enforced by the manipulation of significant sacred symbols and ideas. Subsequently it provokes in all participants a common response, shared meanings and definition of the situation. Through ritual dramas, newcomers (Bucher and Stelling, 1977; Olesen and Whittaker, 1968; Orth, 1963), professionals (Halmos, 1970) and professions (Blankenship, 1977; Larson, 1977) adopt a symbolic-ideological and interactional cloak of competence (Haas and Shaffir, 1977, 1982a, 1982b) convincing outsiders of their competence and trustworthiness in facilitating and easing their crises and status passage.

The methodological appendix at the end of the book provides an account of how the data were collected as well as the methodologically-related problems that accompanied this study. At this point, it is useful to briefly indicate some background concerning the methodology of this work. Our study of the professional socialization of students in the McMaster program involved participant-observation and interview research of a class of 80 students—47 males and 33 females—over a three-year period. From 1974–1977 we observed the students in the full range of their educational experiences, including tutorials, clinical-skills groups, clerkships, and informal gatherings. Our observations recorded as fieldnotes began with the school's admission process for our cohort and continued until the completion of their licensing examination at the end of the third year. Initially the research team consisted of 3 researchers but was reduced to 2 during the second year of the study. Informal interviews were tape-recorded with 58 of the 80 students throughout the period of their medical training; 20 of the students were interviewed at least twice, and several group interviews were also recorded. The school's faculty was not interviewed, although the latter's interaction with students were included in our fieldnotes.

# Chapter II

# *The Setting*

In 1964, the Royal Commission on Health Services in Canada recommended the establishment of new medical schools, including at least one to be located in the Province of Ontario. That same year, McMaster University was selected to develop a school of medicine, and the first dean was appointed in 1965. A small nuclear faculty was recruited and it formed the "education committee." In 1966 the "founding fathers," as they came to be known, conceptualized an approach to medical education which today is referred to as "The McMaster Philosophy."

A characteristic common to the members of the education committee was their dissatisfaction with medical education. There existed a perceived need for a more sensible approach to training physicians. It was mainly during a three year period, available for planning groups to define student learning objectives and for coordinating the over-all organization of the medical school, that the innovative features of the medical curriculum were shaped.

McMaster University Medical School has put McMaster at the forefront of innovation in education, particularly medical education. The School has developed a very comprehensive and explicit philosophy integrating pedagogical concepts and methodologies for creating an education based upon individual and group objectives, interests and needs.

Students develop a methodology emphasizing self-evaluation, self-directed learning and problem solving. Our study examines the student behavior in the context of an expressedly radical departure from tradition bound medical education. A brief description suggests some of the more significant features of this new school and philosophy.

There are several innovative features of the McMaster program which depart from the organization of traditional medical schools. Of these, two are especially striking. First, compared to traditional four-year programs, which are in session approximately eight academic months per year, McMaster has a one-month rather than a four-month summer break. Because long summer vacations are eliminated, the school's program is only three years in duration. Second, applicants are accepted to the medical school without a strong pre-medical background. Students from a wide variety of educational backgrounds, including psychology, sociology, anthropology, the humanities, engineering, physics, and mathematics are accepted into the program. Those lacking a science background were initially required to take special courses in these subjects before commencing the medical program. This pre-medical course has since been discontinued. One of the "founding fathers" expressed the rationalization for the discontinuation of this course:

> Such a program forces a career decision on the student at an early stage and tends to give all students a similar background. Furthermore, the degree earned at the end of a designated premedical course may not be particularly helpful to a student who fails to gain entry to a medical school (Spaulding, 1969:660).

The McMaster medical program consists of a range of innovations that, by themselves, are not novel to education. What is particularly innovative about this program, however, "is the combination of these ideas into a single and unified approach and the creation of an administrative arrangement which allows these ideas to flourish" (Neufeld and Barrows, 1974: 1041).

A most significant departure from the traditional curriculum is McMaster's emphasis on self-directed learning. This is intended to encourage the student, with appropriate guidance, to define his own learning goals, to select appropriate experiences to achieve these goals, and to be responsible for assessing his own learning progress. The student is essentially responsible for the design of his own program and the schedule facilitates this independence with a maximum of one optional class-wide event per day. The stated justification for this emphasis is that if physicians are to be able to assess changing health care needs, and be familiar with changing concepts and new knowledge, the skills to do this should be developed in the formative years of medical school learning.

The emphasis on problem-based learning represents an alternative to studying medicine in a sequentially organized way. Through this approach, the student focuses on a problem which he has identified and brings to it all of his previous information and expertise. As he begins to ask questions, issues become defined which require a further information search. In this manner, the student learns that few problems in medicine are completely "solved." The justifications for problem-based learning are summarized by two of the school's educators as follows:

> Since the problems encountered in medicine are primarily those of individual patients, most problem situations presented to the student relate to an individual clinical case. In this way the learning is highly relevant and similar to the methods by which many health professionals learn in real life. There are many advantages to this kind of learning: it contributes to the student's motivation: it encourages active intellectual processes at the higher cognitive levels; it probably enhances the retention and transfer of information; it can be modified to meet individual student needs; it encourages curiosity and systematic thinking (Neufeld and Barrows 1974: 1042).

As a stated goal of the school, the problem-solving approach challenges the assumption of sequential learning. No attempt is made to "cover" particular content areas: instead, the student is exposed to them in relevant problem situations. Rather than knowledge per se, it is the use of information in the solution of the problem that is encouraged.

To help achieve the aims of the self-directed and problem-solving approaches, the learning format at McMaster is the tutorial session in which five students meet with a tutor—a faculty member who acts as both guide and provocateur. During these sessions various problems are presented and the students discuss their solutions. These meetings "provide a forum for group problem-solving where the pooled resources of the group members, in terms of academic training, experience, personality, and perspective are more effective than the sum of individual abilities" (Neufeld and Barrows, 1974: 1044).

Since the McMaster approach to teaching medicine is shaped around self-directed learning whereby the student is expected to assess his own accomplishments with the assistance of his peers and his tutor, evaluation has changed from the traditional format. The emphasis is on the formative evaluation of the student in which "each assessment provides the opportunity for modifying, or 'forming' the student's learning progress" (Neufeld and Barrows, 1974: 1046). During the course of the learning experience the student undergoes frequent assessments by tutors, peers, and faculty staff. At the end of each learning phase there is a summary statement written by the tutor, informed by the student's self-appraisal and the evaluation of the student's peers. The summary statement prepared by the tutor includes a satisfactory or unsatisfactory progress report. Absent at McMaster are the traditional courses, end-of-course examinations, and grades.

An additional important point concerning the curriculum and a significant departure from the common pattern is the introduction, from the beginning, of students into the clinical setting. This is a particularly noteworthy feature of their training. It represents an attempt to relate student learning with patients having real complaints and problems. The school's stress on clinical experience, as a way of learning medicine, is expected to be a significant distinction between Mac graduates and others.

The most important feature of McMaster Medical School is its uniqueness and its claim (effort) to produce a different kind of professional. This uniqueness has given the school an international reputation as an innovative experiment. It is radically different and much more concerned with the social and educational process. The emphasis on tutorial, self-directed learning, clinical experience, problem-solving, group and self-evaluation, etc. are all predicated on an idea of developing graduates with a different orientation to medicine. In brief, they are prepared to be more capable of coping with the changing nature of medicine as a body of knowledge and as a set of expectations about appropriate behavior. It is believed that they will be more sensitive to the psychosocial needs of patients and to problems encountered in the examination of medical problems. Their approach will be much more holistic, providing an understanding that illness, its sources and treatment, is much more than strictly a matter of health. This broader conception includes an emphasis on behavioral science, particularly psychological and sociological areas, which are, in this approach to medicine, incorporated in definitions and "cures" of human illnesses.

## THE CURRICULUM

The program is divided into four phases of unequal length with additional elective periods and other "horizontal" programs spread across the phases (see figure below).

| Year 1 | Year 2 | Year 3 |
|--------|--------|--------|
| | Summer break | Summer break |
| Phase 1 | | |
| | Phase IIIB | |
| | | Phase IV |
| Phase | Elective | |
| | | II |
| Christmas break | Christmas break | Christmas break |
| Phase II | | |
| | Phase IIIB | Phase IV |
| Elective | | |
| | | Revision |
| | | Revision |
| Phase IIIA | Phase IV | |

Curriculum plan. Phase IV includes a 16 week elective period.
*Source*: Hamilton, British Medical Journal, 1976)

### Phase I

Phase I is a multifaceted introduction to the faculty, the medical community and its resources and aims to provide an overview of the structure and function of the body with some introduction to pathological mechanisms (Sweeney and Mitchell, 1975). There are few, if any, lectures. The students' main concentration is focused around biomedical problems raised and explored in small tutorial groups of five or six. For this phase, the tutor is not selected for his or her expertise in any specific academic area, but rather for skills in getting a group to work together and to acquaint students with, and instruct them in, the McMaster method of teaching and learning. During this phase, approximately 15 biomedical problems are made available as a focus for study. Examples used included that of a child who pours boiling water over herself at home, an infant with diarrhea and vomiting, a retired widower with arterial disease of the legs requiring amputation, and a family with a child with Downs syndrome. The situations are usually presented in written form and some are portrayed by simulated patients. A primary objective during this 10 week period is to help students grasp the essential concepts and to help them achieve a proper balance of priorities. It is also during this period that the new medical student begins developing interviewing and clinical skills.

### Phase II (12 Weeks)

The general theme of this phase is the body's reaction to stimuli and to injury. Concentration is mainly centered on concepts of cell biology and general principles of how cells, tissues and the whole organism respond to stimuli. It is divided into five units dealing in turn with inflammation, neoplasia, metabolic homeostasis, ischaemia, and behavior. As in Phase I, explorations of these areas is through the medium of biomedical problems. The problems are chosen to serve as models of fundamental concepts and the expectation is that students are establishing roots upon which their knowledge will grow. Phase II sees the formation of new tutorial groups with new tutors.

### Phase III (40 Weeks)

In Phase III, four units, each of 10 weeks, are occupied with the major body systems. They are: (a) blood, gastrointestinal system, and nutrition; (b) cardio-respiratory system; (c) neuro-science, locomotor system, psychiatry; and (d) renal physiology and electrolytes, reproduction system and endocrinology.

The tutorial groups are changed for each unit. The standard subdisciplines of microbiology, anatomy, pathology, behavioral science, etc., are integrated into the unit through the use of biomedical problems, lectures and demonstrations. The latter two are usually restricted to about four or five a week. In this phase, clinical problems are explored in greater depth with emphasis on the physical and behavioral mechanisms leading to clinical problems.

### Phase IV

Phase IV is a clinical clerkship in which the student begins to take clinical responsibilities for patients, under supervision. While the student is often acting as an intern, the experience is meant to serve as the epitome of problem-based learning. For the first time there is genuine responsibility for a patient who was seen previously as only a theoretical responsibility.

The objectives of this phase relate to the general approaches to clinical problems rather than detailed subspeciality objectives. Nevertheless, the phase is organized in the settings of the individual specialties. Eight weeks are spent in medicine and eight in surgery. Four weeks each are spent in family medicine, psychiatry, obstetrics and gynecology, and pediatrics. Sixteen weeks are designated for elective experience. Almost a quarter of the program then provides an elective experience, wherein students are able to pursue areas of personal interest, strengthen areas of weakness, and explore individual topics in some depth. In addition, students may have clinical experiences in medical settings elsewhere in Canada or abroad.

### Elective and "Horizontal" Programs

The electives' programs are designed to afford an opportunity to create an individual experience. Sixteen weeks in Phase IV and 10 weeks in the preceding phases are elective. Students no longer work in tutorial groups but design and negotiate their program with their supervisor. They pursue areas of proposed interest, strengthen weak areas, study individual topics, dissect cadavers, explore medical settings elsewhere in Canada or abroad, or repeat the clinical experiences of the standard program. Most take some subspeciality subjects such as ophthalmology, orthopedics or dermatology.

In addition to these electives in blocks, there are some additional programs that run concurrently with the rest of the curriculum. All students take the interviewing and clinical skills programs while the rest are elective:

- *The interviewing program* lasts through Phases I and II. Tutorial groups with a preceptor develop skills in talking to people, dealing with difficult patients, and develop an appreciation for the therapeutic advantages of the interview.

- *The clinical skills program* through Phase III develops ability in history-taking and physical examination and is intended to give an added dimension of reality to the clinical problems under discussion.

- *The community physician program* starts towards the end of Phase II. A student is attached for one-half day a week to a family practitioner working in the community.

- *Emergency medicine* is set up to prepare students to handle crisis situations.

## SELF-DIRECTED LEARNING

The approach to stimulating the student to become a self-directed learner for life is an integral feature of tne undergraduate medical program. The McMaster concept of self-directed learner "involves helping students define their learning needs, select appropriate methods of learning, and evaluate their own learning progress" (Neufeld and Barros, 1974:123–124). The student is assisted by the tutor and/or an advisor in organizing and defining these personal goals and judging their relationship to the objectives of the tutorial group as well as to the overall program goals. The rationale underlying the emphasis on self-directed learning is explained as follows:

> If physicians are to be lifelong learners, able to assess changing health care needs and to keep up with changing concepts and new knowledge by adapting their performance accordingly, the skills to do this should be defined and developed in the formative years of medical school training (Walsh, 1973: 722).

Responsible for the design of their own program, bearing in mind his or her responsibilities to the tutorial group, the schedule facilitates independence with a maximum of one optional class-wide event per day. In line with the importance attributed to this learning approach, approximately 25 weeks in the three-year program are designated for electives—individual time when the student may pursue wide-ranging individual interests and need not consider concurrent responsibilities to the tutorial group.

In addition to determining goals and selecting learning experiences, self-directed learning also involves self-evaluation. Students must be able to evaluate themselves so that they know where they are academically, where they are going and, finally, when they have arrived. Self-evaluation is carried out in the tutorial setting and is viewed as a constant and informal process. The student receives feedback about his or her own performance and assesses it in tutorial discussions with his/her peers, tutor. In addition, feedback is received more formally in reviewing a write-up of a problem with the tutor.

# Chapter III

# Crafting a Successful Biography: Admission to Medical School

For aspiring physicians, the critical career stage is to gain admission into medical school—not an easy task. Admission to medical school is tantamount to becoming a physician as very few fail, or drop out. These facts make significant an understanding of the admissions process as perceived by and subsequently dealt with by the applicants.

The admission procedure can be conceptualized as a form of legitimizing process in which successful candidates construct and/or reconstruct activities in order to idealize themselves in the eyes of legitimators who are known to be examining many other eager, ambitious, and well-qualified applicants. The number of available places is few, while, on the other hand, well-qualified candidates are many. Since there is always a large number eager to be chosen, the ones eventually selected believe they must have stood out as exceptionally qualified for assuming the "professed" role. Choice depends on meeting gatekeepers' expectations by communicating the proper combination of ability, motivation, and experience.

The innovative school we studied has developed three stages for assessing applications. The first involves examination of academic and personal qualities. Applicants must submit a transcript showing their previous academic record. In addition a letter, supported by the inclusion of an autobiographical sketch and other information believed to be relevant to realizing their career goal must also be included. The ones who score highest on this first screening are invited to an interview. During this interview they must submit to an evaluation by a team that usually consists of a medical student, a physician, and a member of the community-at-large; this last member is not necessarily a physician. This part of the process requires applicants to participate in groups of five or six, in a fifty-minute tutorial session. This last exercise is designed to assess the candidates' ability to function within a group. Problem-solving abilities are very carefully rated at this stage of the admission process. The files of those who are judged to have managed the interview and the group session most successfully are examined again. This stage sees the selection of the students for the incoming class.

It is worth noting that although admission to McMaster, (like admission to most medical schools) is supposed to be accessible to all, in reality, the search for students is selective when examined in a socioeconomic context. Research amply demonstrates that decision-makers at medical schools share a social class bias about who should be admitted (Coombs, 1978). Generally, potential neophytes are selected from the middle and upper-middle classes. As we will make clear, the anticipatory socialization of children born into this strata of society provides aspirants to medicine with a biography of experience, carefully crafted, to ensure that candidates present themselves as appropriately trustworthy for undergoing the professionalization process.

In talking to students about their attempts to gain admission, we were impressed by the extent of their preparatory efforts. Aspirants to the medical profession are willing to do anything that is deemed necessary to gain admission to appropriate schools.

Many begin the career process during the secondary-school years, organizing their lives around the idea of constructing a dossier of experiences relevant to their strongly internalized career goal. The autobiographical sketches of the student cohort studied, contain impressive lists of activities and experiences. Experience gained in volunteer work, scientific and/or medical research, positions of leadership, honors, awards, travel, are ones common to many candidates. Candidates are sensitive to the requirements of their evaluators. Thus, they include in their autobiographical sketches descriptions of activities that demonstrate considerable past achievement. Also included is information suggesting their suitability for assuming the responsibility of professional preparation.

It was noted that all successful candidates had performed volunteer work. In their autobiographical statements and letters, they describe the personal satisfactions they experienced in this kind of occupational situation. The importance of this particular pre-professional preparation cannot be underestimated: it is tantamount to an obligatory prerequisite. Applicants correctly perceive that the accepted justification, or vocabulary of motives (Mills, 1940) for their future professionalism, neophyte or occupational, must include the idea of service. The ideology of service justifies the profession's and applicant's claim that they be chosen for, and gain the "license and mandate" (Hughes, 1959) for the special responsibilities that trust imposes.

In talking with students about the preparation of their letters we were impressed by their effort to craft one that was "acceptable." Some applicants had consulted with previously accepted medical students. Their letters had been read and they had received advice about how best to impress the readers. Students described the time and care spent writing and rewriting their letters. It was their hope that they would strike just the right balance in demonstrating their suitability for professionalization. Some were even aware of the rating sheets and criteria used by readers and, therefore, organized their letters around these expectations.

The letters then appear for some as critical to reaching the interview stage of the admissions process and can be understood as attempts to appear outstanding in a larger selection of highly qualified and motivated applicants.[1] The letters are perceived as vehicles of self-promotion in the legitimation process.

We conclude this general discussion of the letter-writing process by pointing out those strategies that successful candidates have in common. First, we note the juxtaposition of the notion that medicine is important, both in terms of providing them with personal fulfillment and in meeting an expressed desire to serve others. We also note how applicants attempt to convince readers about their preparation and interest in the "innovative" program and the goals of family, team and community-oriented practitioners. The following section will examine the letter-writing process in greater detail.

## THE ADMISSION LETTERS

The admission letters of the cohort of medical students we studied were differentiated in several ways. One of the most important distinctions noted relates to a statement of when the idea of becoming a medical student emerged. For many, the idea, and activities supporting this career goal, came early. Such applicants used a consistent set of strategies oriented to the end result of gaining admission to medical school, the first but crucial stage of the professional career. The autobiographical sketches of these early aspirants typically reflect a strong pre-medical or science background, participation in many extracurricular activities which include leadership positions, volunteer work, research experiences in hospitals or universities, and, in many cases, extensive travel.

Those who commit themselves early to the idea of medicine as a career are characterized, by a high degree of motivation whereby they attempt to distinguish and separate themselves from other students in high-school and university. Their motivation is generally reinforced with resources which relate to their parents' position in the class hierarchy. Opportunities to advance their candidacy are available because the parents of this category of students provide the "cultural capital" (Bourdieu, 1973) necessary to cultivate an appropriate pre-professional biography. As members of the middle- and upper-middle classes, these students not only have access to an opportunity structure that facilitates their movement to professionalization but, just as importantly, they are actively encouraged to succeed in their goal of entering the profession of their choice by the family.

It would seem that a disproportionately large number of accepted candidates come from the families of physicians. These applicants argue that their close association with physicians provides them with a realistic basis for choosing a career that might, under other circumstances, be idealized. An extreme example of the familial influences on the choice of medicine as a career is expressed in this applicant's letter when she writes:

> Four members of my family, including my father, are physicians, and two more are studying medicine presently. I have, therefore, been exposed to a doctor's responsibilities and priorities all my life.

The class basis of professional recruitment and memberships, (where education replaces property as a marketable commodity) makes it less likely for those lower in the class hierarchy to be accepted without the resources and the wherewithall available to the middle-class; the idea of pursuing a professional or, in this case, medical career is much more difficult to sustain. Middle-class parents support the idea of a professional career, and the children of these families thus have a tangible advantage. Those lower in the class system are disadvantaged in terms of having no access to an available support system, both in a material and a psychological sense. The working- or lower-class youngster who aspires to a professional career is clearly at a disadvantage in terms of his material resources. Concomitantly, the expressed idea is less likely to be supported and viewed as realistic and attainable by the family.

Two students of the class of 80 we studied were representatives of the working-class. Both of these students admitted to experiencing a sense of marginality from others in the class. This marginality was not only rooted in their limited opportunity structure and support system, but also reflected in a lack of exposure to the kinds of interests and values that characterize the middle-class. As bright young men they were able to overcome the relative lack of resources available to other members of the class, yet they still perceived a difference reflected in the life styles and experiences of their colleagues. One of these students noted the subtle differences in anticipatory socialization when he jokingly said: "The hardest thing for me to learn here is the wines and cheeses." His comment is somewhat facetious but it does point out the difference in life experiences that characterize lower- and middle-class upbringing. The interactional nature of professional socialization and professional activity magnifies the importance of social skills and language competency that characterizes the middle-class.

Thus, we note, (with two exceptions) the class we studied were children of parents who provided a support system that facilitated movement to professionalization. The two exceptions, who overcame the handicaps of their inferior position in the social hierarchy, decided relatively late to become physicians. These two had been successful in academic programs that were not pre-medical, and thus had decided to apply to this new program which accepted candidates outside the typical pre-medical stream. They were career-switchers who, like others without the early idea and motivation for a medical career, reinterpreted their interests and biography to fit this new and belated opportunity.

It was noted that aspirants whose commitment to the idea of medicine came late, particularly those who were involved in other professional careers, for example: engineering, law, research, teaching, nursing, social work and veterinary science, face the necessity of reinterpreting their biography. Career-switchers must provide a suitable "vocabulary of motives" (Mills, 1940) justifying the change, in order that they not be viewed as fickle and/or motivated for the "wrong" reasons. In order to provide this vocabulary of motives they must express the notion that their present career is rewarding and that they are successful. However, they argue that the career they have (up to the time of application to medical school) enjoyed is not enough to provide them with adequate personal fulfillment, given that they wish to assume greater responsibility for the well-being of others. Thus many such applicants expressed dissatisfaction with the impact of their work and felt that *only* medicine could provide them opportunities for making a significant contribution to society.

Application letters of the career-switchers testify how they match their experiences with the notion of suitability for professionalization. The following excerpts from their letters suggest the ways that these aspirants integrate what they have done, with what they hope to do in the future:

> The study of nursing has contributed greatly to both my personal and professional development . . . . Nursing education has increased my self-awareness, sensitivity, and humanitarian concern for others . . . . I have learned to view patients as individuals with emotional, social, as

well as physical needs, which must be considered within the context of their families and communities.

My study of engineering has equipped me with the skills of problem-solving—the ability to recognize a problem, to define its parameters, to consider the various solutions, to choose the optimum solution and to carry out the solution.

As I have grown to know my potentials and abilities, it has become apparent to me that the qualities that I seem to have developed and want to develop are not going to be exploited fully in teaching, nor in any other areas I have tried. Therefore, medicine holds the promise of being able to provide the gratification that will result from constantly learning and working with people to find answers to compelling problems. The potentials of medicine to solve these problems should allow me to develop fully all of my own resources.

Although I have been concerned with research for several years now, I do not feel that this would be a disadvantage to me as a medical student. Indeed, I consider that the insight that I have gained into medical problems in research give me a sense of perspective which will enhance and complement my medical education.

Nursing has given me much . . . . However, of late, I have recognized the historical, legal, and institutional limitations accompanying the nursing role, all of which . . . will continue to stifle my potential abilities as a health-care provider. This is why I want to change my role to that of a physician. I want more responsibility for my actions and . . . more opportunities for leadership. I am aware of the time, effort and cross commitments of pursuing a career in medicine are enormous. It will not be easy, but I am willing to give up things in order to meet these commitments. There may be additional problems too because I am female. But I really believe that I can be a good doctor.

As these and other letters of career-switchers suggest, an internal logic is developed to support the move to a medical career. Always the explanation for the change hinges on the expression of lack of personal fulfillment in their present career and a desire to contribute more to society at large.

All the letters, both of early and late deciders, express the idea of service to others. This is worth further comment. Medicine is frequently described as *the* career that most perfectly combines the opportunities for personal satisfaction and, more importantly, personal service. The ideal of service, of course, lies at the heart of the profession's ideology and helps justify a physician's special authority and dominance in serious and morally fateful matters. It is not surprising, then, that aspirants take on the same vocabulary of justifications, claiming that their desire to serve others would be best accomplished in a profession that makes the same claim. Commitment to the ideal of service means that most letter writers link their need for personal fulfillment with a desire to serve others:

> I have also come to realize that my two foremost goals, serving my own needs and those of others are not incompatible . . . . I found this true especially in my experience in teaching and working with students and professors. Medicine is the only career in which I can meet my goals.

> My ambition and motivation to study medicine is the strongest that my being can integrate, and there is no doubt in my mind that the best and most useful and happy fulfillment I can attain is in the caring for the health needs of my fellow man.

> I want a future that is challenging, self-satisfying and productive to myself and others.

> The only profession which I could feel I can satisfy both my desire to care for and show concern for other human beings and my desire to learn about the human body and how it functions, and at the same time contribute something beneficial to the community is medicine.

> I feel strongly that as a physician I can best realize my own potential as an individual and thus, at the same time, do the most good in the world.

It was also noted that all letter writers made the argument that there was a correlation between previous experiences and the "innovative" philosophy and goals of the new school. Applicants made clear that they were well-prepared, that they had been successful in analogous environments where they had enjoyed problem-solving, self-directed learning, and early clinical experiences, etc. This preparation, it was argued, would complement the school's efforts in graduating community-oriented physicians. The following excerpts from letters make these points:

> Why McMaster? First, it is the program that is suited to my academic background, which lacks basic science courses. More importantly, it is the only place where I can develop my integrated approach to medi-

cine. Second, the structure of learning is best suited to my needs. I have had much experience in, and function best, in a tutorial system. Finally, my experiences in Latin America have directed me to a practice in a rural region. McMaster provides this opportunity.

The prospect of attending McMaster Medical School is indeed an exciting one; however, the prospect of serving the community as a doctor is most exciting of all . . . . My first choice is most certainly McMaster, because the existence of small groups and independent learning opportunities provides an educational setting in which I function best.

I feel that McMaster Medical School, with its "people oriented" and "problem-solving" team approach, and innovative kind of medical training, learning environment and philosophy that I, as a student, would most enthusiastically approach and thus flourish in. I say that because I enjoy and do best in situations where self-directed, unstructured learning is required, as in the hospital last summer.

I have waited several years to be eligible to apply to McMaster. I feel very strongly that my goals, interests and abilities are really suited to the kind of program offered . . . . I have no desire to be part of the medical school system which admits that it is limited by size and structure to the training of good technicians as opposed to "concerned and involved" health care workers.

Through my employment experience, I have gained a humanistic approach to dealing with people. After reading the literature from McMaster and visiting the school, I know that my desires would be satisfied there, both in terms of learning and the philosophical aims.

Since the McMaster Medical School advertises itself as specially organized to prepare practitioners for community and family health care, many applicants express parallel interests. The following quotations from letters demonstrate this expressed commitment:

I would like to be involved as a medical practitioner in a clinic which offered varied services to the public. This would include medical, dental, legal and community services performed and supported by a group of conscientious people who were oriented to community needs.

I have applied to McMaster because it is one of the only medical schools which emphasizes the community role of the physician.

I think inevitably my interest will take me to some kind of community work.

My plans are to become a family practitioner, and either to open a private practice or to work in a small clinic. It is my belief that the family practice program is one of the better answers to efficient delivery of health care to the public.

What I really want to be is a family physician, working with others . . . in an effort to care for the 'total' person and to better the coordination, accessibility and continuity of primary care. As a doctor I would attempt to undertake responsibilities as clinician, educator, and researcher, and I would pursue my goals—to cure, sometimes; to relieve, often; and to comfort, always.

The next stage, comprising the interview and the simulated tutorial, is designed to provide the professions's representatives with a first hand look at how well the candidate meets the professional ideal. Once the candidate has successfully present-ed himself via the vehicle of the autobiographical sketch and letter, he must then via the interview and simulated tutorial prove himself fit to become a member of the profession by demonstrating capability of assuming a role that reflects both competence and trustworthiness. This is no mean task; candi-dates, at this stage, must appear outstanding in the face of equally well qualified competition and, at the same time, dem-onstrate that they will conform to gatekeepers' expectations of "fitting in."

## THE INTERVIEW

The interviews and the tutorial sessions take place over 2 week-ends. At this stage, each candidate knows that he/she has reached another plateau whereupon 80 will be selected from a select list of 432 applicants (Mitchell, et al., undated).

Applicants located at, or near, the university are able to visit the school in advance, cultivate contacts and, in general, "learn the ropes" (Geer, et al., 1968) necessary to successfully meet the rigors of the interview and the tutorial process. At one extreme are those we refer to as "medical groupies." These prospective candidates for medical school made considerable efforts to "psych out" the system. They cultivated relationships with people at the medical school, particularly medical students and faculty, seeking to gain advice on how best to meet gatekeepers' expectations. Some managed to obtain assistance in writing the letter and preparing for interview questions.

The "medical groupies" place such a premium on anticipating gatekeeper expectations and the crafting of an appropriate image that outsiders are put in the position of having a distinct disadvantage. Volunteer interviewers and letter readers from the community occasionally had interests beyond the immediate selection of candidates. This happens when the primary concern of persons involved in the selection process, is to use the situation to personal advantage, or to pass on valuable advice to family and/or friends. As a student cynically suggests:

> They're doing it for somebody they know, somebody who's interested and they've got the opportunity to find out more about the system.

Two students comment on the presence of informal sponsorship within the admissions process. They told us:

> Everyone that I've met who's applying pretty well knows somebody in the program, and is dealing with them, or someone who has a really good friend. You're going to find out who's in the program and get a chance to talk to them.

> It's almost like you've got two strikes against you if you don't know someone who's in the system that can give you inside information. It's almost taken-for-granted.

It is common for students and graduates of the program to be approached by friends, and even by strangers, for any help or advice that might be of use in the admissions process. This sort of comment is typical:

> Other people have asked too. 'Will you read my letter over?' or, 'will you help me write a letter?' or, 'will you prep me for the interview?'

As a result of the effort to "psych out" the admissions process students learn the "codewords" and note the sort of personal image that will fit best with gatekeeper expectations. In this respect, the admissions letter and the interview reflect attempts to present an idealized image. An accepted applicant defines the ideal McMaster candidate when she says:

> They want someone that shows sensitivity, definitely sensitivity, and empathy. These are the big words. They've got to come up in your letter and they've got to come out in your interview. They want someone that can prove that they've got self-directed learning techniques that have worked for them, that they function best under that kind of system . . . . Motivation, definitely motivation. They are all key words. But they're looking for, like a certain kind of motivation. They're different towards family medicine . . . . They want to hear you say that you're coming in basically for primary care.

A third year student describes the ideal candidate in relationship to future expectations and responsibilities when she says:

> They know sort of what they're looking for. Not a loud-mouth. Not a braggard. Someone who's got confidence and shows it, but not over-confidence, where you take on too much, always aware of the patient and willing to grab for extra help . . . .

The interview is administered by three person teams, each monitored by admissions representatives behind one-way mirrors. The membership of the interview team typically comprises a physician, a medical student or health professional, and a volunteer representative from the community.

The candidates who anticipate questions often come prepared with answers, but at the same time they attempt to present an image of spontaneity. A student describes the kind of careful preparation some applicant's make and which might accompany his or her carefully projected image of the self:

> First of all, prepare and anticipate almost any question that can be asked. You've got your answer. And it's style again that's important. You don't jump at answering a question if you're pretty sure. If you know whether you've got the right answer, you just sort of stop and you sort of 'wow, you know, what a question,' even though you know you've been thinking about it and you've prepared yourself. You're thinking, and you're, you know, someone that's a thinker, who just doesn't pop and jump. Because if you do, they're gonna nail you. They're gonna nail you to the cross. And so, you think about it. And you present what you're going to say very logically, not super coolly . . . . Show anxiety. Show the problem-solving going on and not jump at things . . . . If you

can make something funny, make something appear humorous under that kind of pressure, that will get you a long way.

Despite the candidates' efforts to prepare themselves for the interview, by rehearsing responses to questions and dressing carefully, each interview involves a delicate sensitivity to the situation. Some prepared scripts have to be modified or aborted and the applicant's skill at extemporaneous performance is critical. A student describes the interview situation when he says:

> It's your responsibility to feel out the interviewers and modify your answers accordingly to their personality . . . . It's very important to check them out and then what you're going to do is basically say the same thing, but putting it across in that different style, which is what they're looking for.

The critical importance of projecting an appropriate image and controlling the interviewers' perceptions and the interview process is summarized by a successful applicant when he says: "as the applicant you have to control the interview, the interviewer, because if you don't, forget it."

It is considered that women applicants face a special set of image problems: they must communicate a sincere commitment to the practice of medicine in the face of a preconception that marriage and motherhood will interrupt their career (Lesson and Gray, 1978; Oakley, 1976). An additional hazard in the admissions situation they must guard against is the possibility that their appearance might jeopardize the selection process. A male student summarizes the different problems of the good-looking and the unattractive female applicant in these terms:

> If she's good-looking, she's got to watch that she doesn't come across as a sleeze, or someone who's using their sex or good looks, and yet they still have to use that to their advantage in a very coy way. If you're not good-looking, I don't think it's an issue, except not to compensate by being aggressive and independent.

## THE SIMULATED TUTORIAL

On the same day that the interview takes place candidates participate in a simulated tutorial designed to evaluate their performance in small problem-solving groups. Applicants are randomly allocated to groups of five or six members, assigned a group leader, and asked to work through two unstructured problem situations in a fifty-minute session. Assessors, seated behind a one-way mirror, evaluate applicants according to their abilities to relate to their peers, to function in a group and to define and respond to issues in the problem situations (Mitchell, et al., undated).

Candidates, aware of the evaluative criteria, face the delicate problem of facilitating the group process while they, at the same time, must try to distinguish and separate themselves from their competitors. These problems, and the adaptations that accompany them, are central to their success in the group evaluative contexts they will face as students. Applicants were therefore observed taking pains to comment favorably on others' ideas while, at the same time, they attempted to extend the analysis, or to contribute a new or synthetic idea. This approach of demonstrating cooperation and support, while subtly distinguishing themselves, is an adaptation that characterizes the whole professionalization experience and lies at the heart of the interactional basis of reputational control and success in professional life.

Once the applicants have completed the interview and simulated tutorial, they must wait for several months when, during a third stage, their scores are tabulated and final decisions are made about compiling the list of successful applicants and preparing a waiting list for the incoming class.

## CONCLUSION

This chapter describes successful applicants' perceptions of and adaptations to the admissions process of an innovative medical school. The school is "innovative" in that, it provides for two kinds of applicants—traditional "academic" candidates and ones with exceptional "personal qualities." The three-stage process includes the traditional submission of grades and refer ence letters, and more innovative features that include the writing of a personal letter and an autobiographical statement, an interview, and finally, participation in a simulated tutorial.

The successful candidates we studied can be characterized as having met gatekeepers' expectations and by having gained admission by carefully crafting an impression of suitability for professionalization. The importance of the letter for communicating suitability, and the somewhat standardized statements in the letters provides evidence that candidates seek to create an application that reflects the school's expressed philosophy. Letter-writers present themselves as specially qualified and prepared to perform well in the innovative program and willing to project an appropriate professional image. The ideas of personal fulfillment and service to others are revealed as the shared bases of motivation for medicine as a career.

Those who are successful at the letter-writing stage are invited to an interview and simulated tutorial which places a premium on interactional skills and impression-management. In these contexts the applicants attempt to carefully control the impressions others receive of them by standing out from their competition, but not to the extent that they are perceived as having a problem in their ability to conform to professional expectations. Some students cultivate relationships with individuals at the medical school as they seek advice and information on how best to "psych out" the admissions process.

In sum, we note that from the very beginning of the career process, aspirants to the medical profession attempt to manipulate and control others' impressions of them. Legitimation in the pre-professional, professionalizing and professional career involves demonstrating one's credibility before important audiences. As we will see, the strategies used by successful candidates during the admissions process continue to be critical for success in later stages of their career.

# Chapter IV

# *Anxiety:*
# *A Ritual Ordeal*
# *of Professionalization*

Student anxiety and uncertainty are factors common to many studies of socialization into various professions (Bucher and Stelling, 1977; Lortie, 1968; Mechanic, 1962; Olesen and Whittaker, 1968, Orth, 1963), but this is especially true of medicine (Becker et al., 1961; Bloom, 1973; Coombs, 1978; Fox, 1957; Fredericks and Mundy, 1976; Merton et al., 1957; Simpson, 1972). In becoming members of the medical profession, students experience ritual ordeals of uncertainty (Lortie, 1968; Haas et al., 1981) and perceive that professionalization involves their successful taking on of a symbolic role that meets others' expectations.

Professionalization, it is suggested, involves the moral and symbolic transformation of a layperson into an individual who can take on the special role and status claimed by the professional—a process that Davis (1968) labels "doctrinal conversion." In order for individuals to make such significant status changes, they must undergo public initiations or rites de passage that prepare them for the adoption of their new role. A would-be professional must undergo a process of mortification, of testing and ritual ordeal before he/she can be elevated to the special status and role afforded by a profession. This ordeal is important to the professionalization process because it, on the one hand, fosters an image of participants having worked to achieve special competence, and, on the other, because it mirrors the required professional image. Renée Fox (1957) aptly

35

refers to the neophyte's problem as one of "training for uncertainty."

The theme of anxiety that characterizes the uncomfortable adaptation to uncertainty is especially common in reports of research done on groups of medical students (Becker et al., 1961; Bloom, 1973; Coombs, 1978; Fox, 1957; Fredericks and Mundy, 1976; Merton et al., 1957; Simpson, 1972). Doctors do, after all, deal directly with matters of life and death, and their clients often compound this problem by demanding that doctors display authoritativeness, sometimes even casting physicians into the role of demigods.

To demonstrate how professionalization becomes an ordeal for neophytes, we note its central feature: socializers create dramas intended to convince participants and legitimating audiences that the conversion experience is both serious and successful. This belief is typically communicated through ritual mortification processes involving suffering and degradation which convert neophytes into a new and select category of moral persons. The professionalization process (Haas and Shaffir, 1980; Kamens, 1977), like the deviance process (Goffman, 1963; Garfinkel, 1956), involves dramatic rituals which symbolize the transformation of the "called" into "the chosen."

In studying the professional socialization of the McMaster students, we sought to identify the pertinent sources of anxiety and uncertainty they encounter within the program to see if, and how, their methods of coping with them constitute professionalization or the successful negotiation of rites de passage. We also sought to determine if this initiation is different from, or similar to, that which students undergo in traditional programs.

The literature suggests that certain sources of anxiety and uncertainty are likely to be common to all medical socialization settings. The nature of medical education, and the medical profession itself, demands that students perceive the need to be highly concerned about the following factors: internalizing a massive amount of information (including an extensive and highly technical new vocabulary) in a short period of time; avoiding making errors in diagnosis and prescription when they have this responsibility; developing awareness of the imperfect nature of medical science; performing intimate physical examinations, and last but not least, the task of adjusting to the varied reactions of family, friends, and medical faculty and staff to their new medical-student status.

We were not surprised to find that the students we studied, like students in traditional settings, worry about all these matters. We also observed that several of the innovative aspects of the McMaster program cause heightened anxiety in students. For example, students in traditional programs do not conduct physical examinations until the last weeks of their second year. In contrast, McMaster students have contact with patients in the initial stages of the program. Although this innovation provides them with early practical clinical experiences they begin with virtually no guidelines for enacting the qualified and experienced physician's role and thus they are uncertain whether to present themselves in this situation as learners or as neophyte physicians. Variations in patient and staff expectations add to their anxiety.

In this chapter we will, in greater detail, describe and analyze how medical students are initiated into their professional culture. We will examine the nature of the ritual ordeal as it is initially perceived and experienced by a first-year class of students at an innovative medical school. We will explore the sources of anxiety experienced in the socialization experience, seeking to describe those which are general to such experiences and those which are peculiar to the innovative school. We suggest that the traumatic and dramatic nature of "culture shock" experienced by students in the early stages of their medical education is not unique to medical students but rather is characteristic of the professionalization process generally. We suggest this feature of professionalization is heightened in medical socialization, because of the morally fateful "life and death" nature of medical work (Freidson, 1970). We note reasons why Aesculapian authority (Siegler and Osmond, 1973) is afforded the physician.

## ANXIETY ABOUT FUTURE RESPONSIBILITIES

The fateful nature of medical decision-making is perceived as a continuous source of anxiety for the medical students we studied. Though students must meet situational demands, particularly that of meeting legitimator (faculty) expectations, these day-to-day difficulties are superimposed on a continuous and often frightening awareness that the role for which they are preparing requires their making decisions which affect life and death.

It is this type of responsibility that differentiates the physician from other professionals in terms of the responsibilities he must assume. Students are, of course, protected from having to make such decisions without supervision, but they know that each day brings them closer to the time when they will have to face making such decisions themselves. This concern dominates their thinking about developing a self-image that projects an appropriate and trustworthy competence. A student summarizes this concern:

> So what happens is there is a great fear involved now. You're made aware far too often . . . that a person's life is at stake and you have to make the decision. So now people are eager to learn not because of the enthusiasm of the course, not because . . . this is fun and interesting, but because your decision is going to influence somebody's life sometime and you better know the answer . . . . (Interview: Spring, third year).

The problem for all students is assessing whether, in fact, they know what they believe they need to know in order to feel, and be, trustworthy when facing serious medical crises. The problem in both traditional schools and in the innovative school we studied is an ambiguity that makes it difficult to decide what is important to know and whether, in fact, what is known is known well-enough. The problem is exacerbated by the students' realization that in both contexts, evaluation techniques are not always applicable to the problems they will face in real situations. The emphasis on interactional evaluation in the innovative school, and paper and pencil examinations in the traditional school, both serve to contribute to student unease about their ability to predict their future performance. A McMaster student summarizes this general concern about interactional evaluation and future responsibilities when he says:

Of course the medical student doesn't have to know. He does but it's pretty easy to hide. There are some students who don't know much more probably than when they came in and they've been able to hide it pretty well. The danger is that when you're licensed as doctors, . . . we're really licensed to kill people (Interview. Fall, third year).

Students' concern about the validity of whatever type of evaluation they experience, and the problem of assuming responsibility in life and death matters, is amplified by the imprecise nature of deciding what it is that is important to know in the face of the vast amount of information they are called upon to internalize.

### *Learning Massive Information: Too Much To Know*

Studies of medical socialization describe how students in a four-year traditional program face the problem of not being able to study all that is presented to them (Becker et al., 1961; Bloom, 1973; Coombs, 1978; Simpson, 1972). Consequently, students collectively attempt to determine what is important to learn, which usually means knowing the areas on which they will be examined. As the students' immediate problem is to pass examinations and courses, they learn what is likely to be on their examinations. Faced with this problem students develop a short-term perspective—learning what they judge is important to the faculty.

In addition we also observed an anxiety among students about their ability to absorb and integrate such massive amounts of material. The following students' remarks indicate the importance of the problem and the intensity of the anxiety:

There is no way that you are going to be able to learn everything. I mean, there is just an incredible amount of information that is available. I mean, let's face it, there is a fantastic amount that is thrown at you and then the question is 'what are you going to do with all of that, how are you going to tackle that?' . . . the greatest source of anxiety is that there is just a hell of a lot that you have to pick up and that can really make people very neurotic because you know you are trying to learn things, and you realize that there is more to know and so you spend more time learning things and when you learn more things you realize that there is even more to know, and so on. This place can really drive you crazy (Interview: Spring, first year).

I was just telling Vic that the real problem around here is not learning things, but the problem is trying to remember them. I don't think there is anyone around here who has trouble learning things, it's really easy stuff to learn one bit at a time. It's when you have to put it all together, or come back to it two weeks later, and use it that it can be a problem (Field notes: Spring, first year).

The problem around here is not learning, it's forgetting. I don't think there is anyone who has problems actually learning the material, but there is a great deal of concern with trying to remember it (Field notes: Spring, first year).

It's very difficult to see a symptom once, or to examine a patient one time and then to remember what symptoms you observed and what the problem with the patient was. But I find it's impossible to remember. There is just too much stuff that you're trying to remember and you just can't do it, . . . like I can read something over one time and then I'll go back to it and reread it a second time and . . . . I think I'll always remember it. And then when it comes up in a tutorial, it's like I never even heard about this problem before (Interview: Fall, second year).

Unlike the traditional medical school, McMaster de-emphasizes lectures and lacks a formal examination and grading system. Therefore, the problem of having "too much to know" is compounded by the absence of tests and grades which typically serve as standards by which students can measure their progress, particularly when comparing themselves with members of their cohort (Becker et al., 1968).

## THE ABSENCE OF BENCHMARKS

A source of uncertainty created by the innovative approach is the absence of tests and grades. Studies of students in traditional programs (Becker et al., 1961; Bloom, 1973; Coombs, 1978; Fox, 1957; Simpson, 1972) show that they generally face the problem of absorbing massive amounts of information by attempting to determine, collectively, what it is that is important to learn. Since their immediate goal is to pass examinations and courses, they study that which they deem relevant to the faculty and hence likely to be on their examinations. Typically, they then use their grades as standards for assessing their progress by comparing themselves with members of their class. Since the McMaster program includes no grades or examinations, the students have no clear benchmarks of progress, which compounds their dealing with the problem of having "too much to know."

The students are, of course, evaluated regularly and frequently. In one type of evaluation, students must do write-ups of problems, which their tutors read and review. Members of each tutorial group are also called upon to assess each other's progress, competencies, and inadequacies. This form of evaluation produces much anxiety because few, if any, students have had to reveal so much of themselves in previous educational contexts. Moreover, the overall picture of individual progress remains unclear because each student has only his or her tutorial group as a reference.

Some students said they favored the traditional educational methods to which they were accustomed. In earlier educational experiences they had experienced a measure of security by passing tests and by competing successfully with other students. After all, their earlier success with these methods was one of the important determinants of their being selected out of a vast number of applicants. In the innovative program on the other hand, there are no clear benchmarks of progress. The relationship of uncertain progress and student anxiety is expressed by the following students' comments:

> I think a lot of people would like to have tests and grades and then they would be able to measure themselves and also they would feel confident that they are done with an area and they could leave that behind. They've learned enough about that. That is one of the problems we have is never knowing if we learned enough. With tests and grades that problem might be better resolved. That is why people are anxious, they don't really get the feedback as to whether they do know enough (Interview: Spring, first year).

> You know it's kind of like an initiation and they keep it like that . . . . So part of it is to humble you. They sure do a good job of that. They don't really tell you where you are weak and where you are efficient. All your evaluations are generally favorable and so you don't have a real sense of how you're doing. If there was some way of better knowing whether

you are doing well or not, it would be very, very helpful (Interview: Spring, first year).

Although students do not take conventional tests and thus do not have to complete for grades, teachers regularly and frequently evaluate them. In one type of evaluation, student write-ups of problems are submitted to tutors for reading and review. In another important, nontraditional form of evaluation, members of each tutorial assess each other's progress and contributions and analyze their own progress, competencies, and inadequacies. This innovative form of evaluation initially produces high levels of anxiety, because, as has already been noted few, if any, students have had to reveal themselves in this way. Two students make this point by saying:

> The biggest difference for me here, is that you have to reveal more of yourself. You can't hide yourself. You're open to scrutiny and you expose yourself in the tutorial as part of your education (Field notes: Winter, first year).

> You know, I think you have to have a lot of confidence as a group to go through what we're going through now (evaluation). I mean you're opening yourself up to peoples' comments, to their criticisms and it's really like pulling down your pants (Field notes: Winter, first year).

The educational system in which these students were previously successful, afforded them a protective cloak of anonymity. At McMaster, students' personal evaluations are supposed to reflect candor and include "confessions" of guilt and rededication to their education and student colleagues. The following, based on observation of a tutorial group evaluation, illustrates how students manage this problematic situation:

> It was time for the students' evaluation and it was clear that no one knew exactly how to go about it. Tom (tutor) offered, 'Oh why don't we bad-mouth the tutor and start from there?' Alex said, 'I'd be willing to go first, what do we want to do? Do we want to all talk about each other or have Tom talk about us first or what?' Gerry said, 'I've already filled in the evaluation form on myself. What I would like to do is go through it with you and you tell you my own analysis and the scores that I gave myself and when I'm done then we could comment on my impressions and whatever evaluations you have, and then maybe I could revise these scores that I've given myself (Field notes: Winter, first year).

What we find noteworthy in this example (and in other evaluation situations observed) is that students approach the evaluation process with great caution. Students often try to do the evaluation in a setting familiar to them or to turn some of the session into a "social occasion." In the previous excerpt, we can interpret Gerry's suggestion for the evaluation procedure as his attempt to retain a high degree of control over his own evaluation. We see him attempting to control participants' definition of the situation.

Students have little to gain by challenging self-praise, and little incentive to criticize their peers. While evaluations are supposed to be critical, they become in the end, teamwork efforts (Goffman, 1959) in which each student tacitly agrees to be "nice" in order to collectively produce an overriding sense that everything is going reasonably well. Ironically, this "gentleman's agreement" increases private doubts about progress because the individual compares him/herself to the common judgment that everyone is doing well. Tutorial evaluation often creates a situation of pluralistic ignorance (Schanck, 1932:102, 130–131; Mayer and Rosenblatt, 1975) whereby students avoid negative evaluation that violates the "gentleman's agreement," choosing rather to suggest that everyone is doing well. In a situation having such unclear standards, and measures of progress and competence, we observe both students and tutors avoiding a confrontation that will disrupt the collective commitment to reducing the threat of making truly critical judgments. A situation develops where severe criticism might reverberate throughout the institution thus making all participants vulnerable to direct attack. Privately, students and others are criticized, but mainly through gossip, which does not disturb the shared commitment to the developing of an harmonious situation. This, we contend, is the main reason why students choose to make only individual responses to the anxiety they experience in the early months of their training. They role play and attempt to control others' impressions of them by adopting a symbolic-ideological "cloak of competence" (Haas and Shaffir, 1977).

Group evaluation, then, provides only an imperfect indication of the student's mastery of medicine, with his or her own tutorial group taken as a reference group. They face the additional problem of estimating the competence of their own tutorial group in relation to that of other tutorial groups. This situation is aggravated by the prevailing notion that it is considered inappropriate to visit other tutorial groups for comparative purposes. Students therefore compare themselves and their group to others only on the basis of rumor and informal conversation.

## TRAINING FOR UNCERTAINTY

As students progress, they are immediately confronted by the complexity of the subject matter of medicine. They learn that it is difficult to keep abreast of new discoveries and advances in the medical sciences, and, more significantly, that medicine is an imperfect science. Renée Fox aptly summarizes this important source of student anxiety when she characterizes medical student socialization as "training for uncertainty":

> Students were confronted with three basic types of uncertainty as they advanced from one phase of the curriculum to another: (1) uncertainties that stem from the incomplete mastery of the vast and growing body of medical concepts, information, and skills; (2) those that come from limitations in current medical knowledge and techniques; and (3) the uncertainties that grow out of difficulties in distinguishing between personal ignorance or ineptitude and the open-ended, imperfect state of medical science technology, and art (Fox, 1974:202).

When discussions in tutorials turn into unsettled debates and when the accuracy and suitability of patient diagnoses and treatments are seen as problematic, students realize not only that there is too much to learn but also that much will change, or even remain unknown. A student expresses this awareness in Phase II when he says:

> A lot of what we do we know the consequences of but we don't know the processes involved. We don't know what interaction takes place. We just know the end result and we continue to use it because the end result seems favorable. One of the intangibles that we can't measure is how much a patient's desire to improve affects his improvement and how much of medicine or a particular technique helps (Interview: Winter, first year).

The student becomes aware during Phase I, with its heavy emphasis on the psychosocial aspects of health, that environmental and emotional factors are important, but that these factors remain vague and generally indeterminate variables that affect patient well-being. As at other medical schools (Becker et al., 1961, ch. 11; Coombs, 1978; Coombs and Boyle, 1971; Fox, 1957), the ambiguity and complexity of medical science in their clinical experience is perceived as even more profound.

Clinical experience at McMaster begins not in the third year, as is the case in traditional medical schools, but rather in the first few weeks of the program, before many students feel comfortably adequate in regard to their command of necessary medical knowledge. In a clinical practise environment, students begin to appreciate the uneasy relationships between patient symptoms, diagnosis and treatment. They learn first-hand the imprecisions of medical observation and testing in accurately determining the cause(s) of a patient's condition. Simple matters like listening to heart sounds or the taking of blood pressures are not always confidently accomplished. The problematic nature of physical observation of a patient is noted in the following discussion between a student and faculty clinician:

> Harper (student) says, 'You know, I've checked some people's ears, but I'm really not sure that I'm seeing what I'm supposed to be seeing. Sometimes when someone looks into the ear you say: 'Did you see this?' They'll say 'yes' even though they never saw it.' The clinical preceptor says: 'Don't feel too bad about this, because I'm telling you that even when I look into an ear I don't always see what I believe I'm supposed to' (Field notes: Fall, first year).

Besides trying to master a vast and complex body of clinical information, students must learn the highly technical and specialized language of the profession. At this very early stage of their training, the sheer inundation of a new language, and the internalization of a complex medical terminology, confuses students, making it more difficult for them to understand their subject material. They become uncertain about whether they will ever understand and become facile with the communication tools at their disposal.

Learning the language is critical to students' symbolic participation and identification with the profession (Roth, 1957).

For the students, facility with medical terminology is a prerequisite for acceptance and recognition by faculty and peers, and demonstrates, to important others, that they have not only learned knowledge but can apply it.

## ANXIETY FEEDING ANXIETY

A marked change comes over students when they try to achieve standards of learning in an educational system which lacks clear standards. We observed students working day and night, and through weekends, trying to "keep pace" and "cope with" their feelings of uncertainty and anxiety. A student describes how all-encompassing their work becomes when he says:

> I have to spend the weekends working or else I just fall too far behind. I find that you just don't take medicine, you live it. You eat it and sleep it (Interview: Winter, first year).

Ironically, and in contrast to the findings of Becker et al. (1961), their shared perspective incorporates an individualizing, rather than a collectivizing, mode of action. Due to the pressures to appear and become more competent, and the complexity and disputable nature of much of the material, (including the fact that much could be found in books and articles) students in their first year work hard and in private. Unlike the traditional medical school, the innovative school supports and encourages students to learn individually. This is part of the school's philosophy to develop independent doctors who will be motivated professionals for the rest of their lives. Faculty encourage students to consider the learning of medicine as a life-long process, and that early socialization is basic methodological preparation for later independent research and study (Neufeld and Barrows, 1974; Spaulding, 1969).

Teachers and students create a collective support for independent work and, although some of the students' experiences are group and cooperative ones (tutorial and clinical experiences), much of the activity involves a private struggle to learn and absorb medical knowledge. The pressure to appear, and eventually to be competent in the space of a three-year program creates in the students' minds a situation requiring the maximum individual attention. They feel they should not only study hard, but alone.

Because the students isolate themselves from each other, they create a new source of anxiety and insecurity: loneliness. Two students describe the process this way:

> I think we work so hard at it, we really become alienated. I think that one of the problems that most of us have is that we haven't been able to develop real friends here, because we're wrapped up in getting our work done. I think a lot of people feel this. You just don't feel like there is any time to relax, because you always got it hanging over your head (Interview: Spring, first year).

> I think that basically students in the class are very lonely. You know as individuals we don't have the time to really have other relationships outside the class and we are never in a situation where we can meet other people. And you know if the class is not nicely rounded ·out in terms of finding companionship from each other, then it's a difficult situation (Interview: Spring, first year).

Many students feel that they must put interpersonal relationships aside because of the pressures of their learning, and this creates a related insecurity. The students are caught up in a vicious cycle. They become over-anxious when not working hard, because they fear that they are not keeping up and learning enough, and as they attempt to assuage that concern by working hard, they find themselves more and more alienated from their fellow students and friends. The following excerpt reflects this feeling of isolation:

> . . . one of the greatest and saddening features perhaps is the fact that there aren't too many people outside of medicine that I relate to and it's not a consequence so much of my own choice, but it's just the fact that outside of that school the world rarely exists, and I just don't have the time to explore it. That's a really big regret, the fact that people around me are really working very hard and mostly of their own neurosis that they do . . . . They tend to really overwork. This puts you in a position where you too work very hard and you just get caught up in it (Interview: Winter, second year).

Students work hard in an attempt to assuage or relieve their anxiety but they also begin to take on a role and demeanor that provides them with a protective "cloak of competence" from the threat of being defined as incompetent. Students begin, in the tutorial, to learn how to manage themselves in ways that give them control over the situation and lessen the possibility that mistakes or incompetence will be charged or revealed.

### Managing the Medical Student Status

An essentially unreported and neglected issue in studies of medical socialization is the problem medical students face adjusting to their new status. Although an extended period of socialization awaits, admission is virtually tantamount to membership in the profession because few fail to successfully negotiate the training period. Selection, therefore, becomes the crucial stage of status passage and with it, emerge problems of status management (Glaser and Strauss, 1971). Acceptance into a most prestigious and respected profession brings with it an accompanying alteration in status in the eyes of others, and, ultimately, in the mind of the possessor. A student describes this initial reaction when he says:

> I think like you've made it into medical school which is a tremendous boost for the ego and it sort of sets you up so many notches in terms of your own self-confidence, just getting into medical school (Field notes: Winter, first year).

Students often report that their new status of medical student creates difficulties for them in their relationships with significant others. They feel unchanged, but are treated as possessing a markedly enhanced status. A student describes the reactions of others and the problem it creates when he says:

> It is a problem because people immediately think of you as something special, and you don't want them to think of you as something special. It gets to be a hassle (Field notes: Winter, first year).

One of the observers was present when an employee at the medical center was informed of his admission. Needless to say, he was euphoric and his colleagues seemed genuinely pleased. A bottle of champagne and a cake were brought out for a brief, but exuberant, celebration. A female colleague made, perhaps, the most telling comment when she said: "I just hope you don't let medical school go to your head. Try to stay as nice as you are."

The above comment reflects a more generalized reaction to success that acceptees described to us. Many mentioned that their acceptance into medical school initiated a set of reactions that seemed to redefine them as special people. Accepted students are treated with a new respect and deference, commensurate with their new master status (Hughes, 1945) which becomes their primary badge of identity and the major focus of any outside interaction with them. A female student describes the vulnerability of the medical students new identity to such interaction when she reported this about her Christmas vacation:

> It was incredible. Everybody was coming to me for advice. They'd tell me the symptoms and ask me what to do. My grandmother asked me to accompany her to the doctor and on the way back she told me what the doctor said and asked me what it meant (Interview: Spring, first year).

Students find that, more and more, rather than treat them interpersonally, friends and family put them in the structural role of "doctor." They are treated like indigenous medical experts who are related to chiefly on the basis of their new identity and presumed expertise. Within the medical school complex they are typically treated as being of the chosen few. Outside the school, in affiliated hospitals and services, they receive varied reactions. Even within the medical school, their neophyte and subordinate status is reinforced on numerous occasions. More importantly, their own insecurity about how well they are learning medicine and how successfully they are wearing the privileges and prerequisites of their acclaimed status, have important anxiety-producing effects despite the deferential and isolating or elevating reactions of others. They live with the knowledge that they are not all that is expected of them, bearing the burden of living up to a standard that no one can accurately measure.

### The Patient as a Source of Anxiety

Because McMaster medical students deal with patients at an earlier time than students in most other schools, they have less of an introduction to medical science to guide them and allow them to properly enact a professional, physician-like role. They receive no clear guidelines about whether to emphasize the learner, or the student-physician role. Although students are introduced to patients as students, we observed a range of demeanor with patients that indicated students were not consistent in emphasizing either part of their role. While this innovation of the school provides students with practical clinical experiences, the ambiguity of their role and the variations in patient and staff expectations adds to their anxiety.

Students begin by taking patient histories and eventually move on to doing physical examinations. We found that initially the physical examination was the most anxiety-producing aspect of their contact with patients. This supports Fox's (1974:206) finding:

> Certain aspects of the history and physical were particularly embarrassing and emotion-laden experiences for students; for example taking a sexual history; examining a woman's breast; doing a vaginal or pelvic examination, palpating a man's testicles or a person's abdomen; carrying out a rectal examination. These intimate and potentially erotic aspects of the clinical tasks they were learning to perform, along with 'any very emotional reaction' by a patient were likely to be disturbing to students. For, at this point in their training, most students were struggling to manage their own over-abundance of concerned feelings and to achieve greater detachment as they undertook their still very new, physician-like role.

We observed that students varied in their confidence about the problem of sexuality when examining patients. At one extreme was a student who attempted to alleviate the anxieties of her fellows by allowing herself to be examined:

> When we took the clinical in Phase I, we used to listen to each others' heart sounds and all four of the guys each week took off their shirts and allowed us to listen to them and palpate them. I thought it would be kind of inevitable that a girl would do it. But I knew that the guys were nervous about it so we started talking about it in tutorial. I decided that it is kind of foolish. I mean it's only a human body, and I would volunteer because I didn't think the other girl should do it. So I volunteered to let them do a breast examination. I told Dr. James, I believe he's kind of a blue-nose. I think he was shocked by it. It didn't bother me and I thought it would be a good experience for them. So I did it. I let them

examine me, and I wasn't bothered at all. I'm sure they were bothered, at least initially, but after a time I noticed that they seemed to be able to deal with it more objectively (Interview: Winter, first year).

For most of the students, however, examining patients of the opposite sex produces a different response to anxiety:

When Dr. Michelson [clinical skills preceptor] was out of the room, a medical student, says: "It's happened again, another beautiful woman. I didn't do an examination. I walked in and I saw how beautiful she was and I just put my hands in my pockets." He put his hands in his pockets demonstrating how he'd tried to act professionally. When Dr. Michelson returned, Joe [the student] told him that Lawrence has said he was nervous because he had another beautiful patient. Dr. Michelson smiled and asked: "You didn't examine her then?" Lawrence replied: "No, I didn't have time. I guess I'll try and do it this evening" (Field notes: Winter, first year).

A student about to examine a simulated patient says, "I hear that they really picked a beauty for this. Like she's really supposed to be a sharp babe. So I don't know how it's going to be in there." After the exam, he says with a smile, "She really is a sharp-looking babe. I would've liked to do a lot more with her but you know, under the circumstances, it would really have been improper" (Field notes: Winter, first year).

Examining patients, particularly those of the opposite sex, is a shared student problem that is perceived with uncertainty and discomfort. This is particularly true of students in the early phases of their training where they have not yet learned how to control themselves or their patients.

Students' anxiety about examining patients' sexual parts remains, but they gradually limit and control it through carefully managed performances. Students try to conceal their nervousness and discomfort, which they partly manage, by adhering to the ritual of draping patients' sexual parts. Students effect a serious and professional posture with patients in order to turn a potentially erotic or embarrassing situation into a clinical one (Emerson, 1970). A successful performance is one in which the patient is comfortable, thereby allowing the student to relax.

Also, students feel they are expected to act as cooly and objectively as some of the practitioners they observe. Students criticize these doctors for being "insensitive" or "callous" to patients. As the students move towards an attitude of "detached concern" (Merton, 1957) they fear that they will not strike the appropriate balance of detachment and concern. In moments of idealism, students believe that they will not act impersonally towards their patients; at the same time they recognize that the demands of socialization may corrupt them (Fox, 1974; Coombs and Boyle, 1971).

## CONCLUSION

A significant part of professionalization is an increased ability to perceive and adapt behavior to legitimators' (faculty, staff, and peer) expectations, no matter how variable or ambiguous they are in nature. Medical students in both traditional programs and the innovative program we observed are uncertain about the relevance of their curricula to the demands they will face as professionals. Both groups are also dubious about the effectivness of their respective evaluation processes. In this context of ambiguity, students in both settings accommodate themselves, individually and collectively, to convincing others of their developing competence by selective learning and by striving to control the impressions others receive of them.

The innovative professional setting that we studied differs in curriculum and pedagogical methods from traditional medical schools. Yet these differences do not seem to alter the character of the ritual ordeal that students experience. In both settings, students must accommodate themselves to uncertainty. They do this by selective learning and a careful presentation of self. We conclude that the different organizational structures serve the same purpose: they provide and dramatize the ritual ordeal of students, thereby legitimating the idea that important changes have taken place. The ordeal character of the socialization process communicates, to established professionals, outsiders, and the students alike, the exceptionality of the conversion experience and the development of trustworthy competence.

# Chapter V

# *Becoming Professional: Learning and Adopting A Cloak of Competence*

In his seminal work on social interaction, Goffman (1959) draws attention to the significance of impression management in everyday life. In order to explore this dimension of social life, sociologists have focused mainly on people involved in deviant and low status occupations (Ball, 1967; Edgerton, 1967; Goffman, 1961; Henslin, 1968; Maurer, 1962; Prus and Sharper, 1979; Scott, 1968). Yet as Hughes (1951) suggests, a comparative study of occupations often reveals similar adaptive mechanisms. In occupations that demand a measure of trust from clients, participants must convince legitimating audiences of their credibility. The importance of playing an adequate role in order to exact the right kind of response from clients is true of both shady and respectable occupations.

Although impression management and role playing are essential parts of this kind of sociological interaction, effective performance becomes even more crucial when participants perceive an audience that is potentially critical and condemning. This is especially true when an audience has high expectations of competence in others. If those in whom competence is expected also have a concomitant responsibility of making decisions that affect the well-being of others, the situation is even more crucial. Audiences then look for cues and indications of personal and/or collective (institutional) competence and in response practitioners organize a carefully managed presentation of self intended to create an aura of competence.

Concern about the competence of those granted rights and responsibilities affecting others is very much a part of the relationship existing between patients and medical professionals. Patients look for competent advice and assistance and medical professionals, particularly doctors, want to convince those they treat that they are indeed competent and trustworthy. It is only when a patient believes a doctor possesses these attributes that diagnostic intervention and prescribed treatment can affect the course of the illness in any positive way.

Studies of professional socialization (Becker et al., 1961; Bloom, 1973; Broadhead, 1983; Light, 1980; Merton et al., 1957; Olesen and Whittaker, 1968; Ross, 1961) show how trainees adopt a professional image as they proceed through the socialization process. Sociological studies of noncollege, school and other training situations (Geer, 1974) indicate that the socialization experience involves learning specific skills and techniques as well as taking on an occupational culture which includes a new or altered identity. Such studies describe a process whereby students or trainees adapt in order to develop a new view of the self.

As students are professionalized, they are initiated into a new culture wherein they gradually adopt those symbols which represent the profession and its generally accepted authority. These symbols (language, tools, clothing, and demeanor) establish, identify and separate the bearer from the outsider, particularly from the client and the paraprofessional audience. Professionalization, as we observed it, involves the adoption and manipulation of symbols and symbolic behavior which creates an imagery of competence. The net result of this process separates the profession from those they are intended to serve.

Faced with inordinately high audience expectations, medical students begin the process of professionalization by distancing themselves from those they interact with. They manipulate the symbols of their new status in order to distinguish their activity as one grounded in mystery and sciences unfathomable to others. Their performance is intended to convince both themselves and others that they are competent and confident to face the immense responsibilities imposed by their privileged role.

This chapter will demonstrate the ways in which the medical students we studied attempted to communicate trustworthiness by impression-management. The focus is mainly on the clinical, or clerkship experience, this being the critical phase of the ritual ordeal where the professionalization process is most intense. We begin by outlining the general expectations that delineate the physician's role and the perceived expectations of the student in clinical training. Then we describe the importance of the manipulation and control of people, symbols, and ideas that is necessary for meeting both generalized and situational expectations. We especially note the specific problems involved in the process as perceived by students in the innovative program.

As students become successful at controlling and manipulating others' impressions in order to be perceived as competent and trustworthy, they increasingly identify with the role and with the ways that qualified practitioners handle their problems. Successful control of professionalizing situations, it would seem, has a self-fulfilling quality which allows authoritative performances to contribute to the neophytes' changing perceptions of the self. If initiation is rigorous, students learn to adopt a symbolic-ideological cloak of competence that they perceive initiated members of the medical fraternity to wear. It is thus that the image of authority and trustworthiness is created. By way of a conclusion we will point out that the nature of legitimating audience expectations are perceived by newcomers as requiring conformity to a role that is exaggerated and thus demands an exaggerated performance.

## GENERALIZED EXPECTATIONS OF COMPETENCE

The medical profession is a unique one in that so much of its authority depends on the effective communication of trust. Freidson (1970:10–11) outlines the characteristics of this occupation that serve to set it apart from others. These are:

- A general public belief in the consulting occupation's competence, in the value of its professed knowledge and skill.
- The occupational group . . . . must be the prime source of

the criteria that qualify a man to work in an acceptable
fashion.

- The occupation has gained command of the exclusive competence to determine the proper content and effective method of performing some tasks.

Medicine's position, Freidson (1970:5) notes, is equivalent to that of a state religion: "... it has an officially approved monopoly of the right to define health and illness and to treat illness."

Doctors possess a special authority because of their accepted expertise about human health. Their work is believed to constitute a social and individual good. Their authority is further enhanced by the historical linking of medicine and religion: the physician mediates the mysteries of scientific research through a ritual system where the doctor assumes a priest-like role (Siegler and Osmond, 1974:42).[1]

To create a physician's authority requires the manipulation of an effective symbol system which is accepted and shared by participants. The moral authority of the physician is most apparent as being complete and unassailable when the doctor is involved with decisions affecting life and death. The fact that death strikes fear in human beings gives impressive, Aesculapian authority to those who are believed able to ward it off or postpone it (Siegler and Osmond, 1973).[2]

Because of the authority invested in them, medical practitioners, students and physician alike, must deal with the inordinate and exaggerated demands of those they treat. The problem is somewhat less in magnitude for the medical student, who is generally protected from situations which would prematurely or inappropriately demand his exercise of inappropriate responsibility. Students, however, realize that the outcome of their socialization will, in the future, require them to deal with life and death situations. It is thus their hope that the socialization process will prepare them to meet the responsibilities imposed by their profession with both confidence and competence. According to one student:

> I think you're faced with a problem, that in a large way the public has
> unrealistic expectations about the medical profession. It puts the doctor

in a very difficult position because you know yourself you don't know it all, but the public thinks you know it all and puts you in a position where you have to be a good actor (Interview: Winter, second year).

### The Problems of Perceived Expectations in Clerkship

During the rotating clerkship assignments, the students are exposed to many different audiences which all have different expectations about the proper performance of the role. In fact, in the hospital setting, the role itself is ambiguous and raises the question, is the individual primarily student, clerk or physician? As a result, the 'clinical jerk' is constantly faced with new situations that do not relate in a clear way to his new status. In consequence he finds it difficult to assume an appropriate role and to project a "correct" identity.

Another confusing aspect of the clinical clerk's situation concerns the responsibility he/she is expected to assume. In earlier phases of the program the student examined patients as part of a learning experience; clerkship demands that the students do more than learn. He must assume a degree of responsibility for patient well-being. A student summarizes this difference when he says.

Well, from my perception, even in Phase II and Phase III, we played around with real patients in a Phase I sort of thing . . . . It was sort of a game. You were trying to find out what was the interesting clinical sign. Whereas now (clerkship) when you see a patient you are doing a history and physical on a patient and it sort of focuses on you . . . . The intern may or may not go over the bloody patient because he's really trusting you to pick up what you should pick up . . . so you're always trying to think, 'Well, if I don't pick these up, and the resident doesn't get them, I'm the one who has done the history and physical. If I miss something, then somebody is going to be after my ass for it' (Interview: Winter, third year).

As students in clerkship become more integral members of a health care team, they are delegated some tasks which require the exercise of personal responsibility, and thus they become accountable in ways almost always new to them. The taking on of increased responsibility and the concomitant exercise of medical judgment makes them accountable to a variety of professionals. The prevalent response of the clinical clerk is to develop an increasingly sympathetic attitude towards their future profession. The following examples gleaned from clinical clerks illustrate this point:

> (The conversation centers around clerkship and whether this phase of the program alters one's view of the medical profession.) I think it does from the point of view that you can more or less see other peoples' situations much more because you're in their boat. . . . Having been in it (medicine), I can see why some patients are dealt with quickly perhaps (Interview: Spring, second year).

> I remember when we were way back in Phase II and Phase I, we would go see a patient with a clinical skills preceptor, and he might have said something to the patient that seemed rude, and I'd get all very indignant about it and say: 'My God, you're not being sensitive.' While that may have been justified, now that I'm on the ward I can see that in a way it's a bit silly to take that one episode, because what you are seeing is one episode in a long history of the relationship between that patient and his doctor. You're taking this totally out of context and it's really not relevant to criticize unless you really know the relationship. Now I'm much less free with those sorts of criticisms (Interview: Spring, second year.

Students are confronted with a dilemma. On the one hand they try to prove themselves as competent to others, while on the other, they remained concerned about the limits of their competence which might cause them to act inappropriately, perhaps with dire consequences. Two students summarize this ambiguous response to the taking on of responsibility this way:

> Jim complains to Claudette that on one of his rotations he was given too much responsibility. He says, 'I don't mind it if I'm ready for it, but I just didn't feel I was ready for it. The resident thought I was ready for it. He thought I knew more than I did. Maybe I did, maybe I didn't. If I did, I suppose I was ready for it, but I didn't feel I was ready for it. I didn't feel I knew enough but he tells me I knew enough. I felt uncomfortable and asked that I not be given the responsibility' (Field notes: Spring, third year).

### Adaptations to Interactional Evaluation

While students are generally protected from meeting all the expectations of patients, they do face the unpredictable nature of faculty expectations; in fact, faculty become the major reference group or audience that students feel most demand and evaluate competence. The teaching staff is responsible for evaluating and determining the progress of the students. The students, in turn, attempt to estimate teachers' demands, although at times they are ill-defined and sometimes contradictory. Defining and attempting to meet faculty expectations is often difficult. The students' problem is dealing with staff who have widely divergent approaches to the practice of medicine. Faced with a threatening ambiguity, students try to find out the particular biases and special areas of interest of those with whom they must interact (Becker et al., 1961). This is because they soon realize that their teachers are convinced of the correctness and validity of their expertise and approach. In this sort of situation the students find their competence and learning assessed in situations in which they are vulnerable and therefore easily reminded of their incompetence.

For professional students the short-term goal of a "good" evaluation is vital because this kind of assessment demonstrates their developing competence to those who control their careers. To a lesser extent this is also true of students in traditional medical-school settings. Although these students initially impress the faculty by their skill at passing examinations, they must eventually demonstrate competence. This is similar to students in the innovative program, through the exercise of selective interactional skills. Both types of students, those in traditional and innovative learning environments, then exhibit a common reaction to evaluation in the face of uncertain expectations. When individuals are uncertain about what they should know or how they should apply it, they "cover" themselves by deflecting others from probing their ignorance (Edgerton, 1967; Goffman, 1963; Haas, 1972, 1977; Haas and Shaffir, 1977; Olesen and Whittaker, 1968). This "cloaking" behavior is often accompanied by initiative-taking behavior intended to impress others with their competence. This phenomenon is well-documented. For example, Becker et al. state:

> Perhaps the most noticeable form of attempting to make a good impression is the use of trickery of various kinds to give the appearance of knowing what one thinks the faculty wants one to know or having done

what the faculty wants done, even though these appearances are false (1961:284).

Bucher and Stelling also report that students, themselves, are aware that impression management is crucial to their progress.

> The residents have learned that *they* could contribute considerably to the nature and outcome of the supervisory process. . . . The most common tactic was that the resident psyched out what the superior wanted to hear and presented his material accordingly (1977:107, 109).

Since the students in the tutorial-based program we observed write no formal examinations, they learn to handle interactional evaluation much earlier than their peers in traditional programs. As one student observes:

> One of the pressures that people probably meet when they come in here is that in tutorial learning not only does your learning center around the tutorial group but your evaluation centers around your performance in the tutorial group. It's very beneficial to be the type of person who functions well within a group, not necessarily as a bright or intelligent person, or even one who knows his stuff, but one who functions well within groups. In the class there is a lot of pressure to be that kind of person. . . . (Interview: Spring, third year).

Most are critical of the approach. Their objections, which range from mild concern to severe criticism, do not center on any particular complaint but includes a variety of considerations.

Especially during the early stages of the program, many students express a desire for some kind of testing or "objective" evaluation to ease feelings of uncertainty.[3] One student sums up:

> I think a lot of people would like to have tests and grades and then they would be able to measure themselves and also they would feel confident they are done with an area and they could leave that behind. . . . That is one of the problems we have—never knowing if we learned enough (Interview: Winter, second year).

In addition the students we studied are, generally, concerned about the validity of the process of self- and group-evaluation in the tutorial groups. Consensus has it that the participants anticipate a "gentleman's agreement" and they collectively collude to assess each other positively. A third year student's comment illustrates this concern:

> I think the evaluation system is . . . inadequate. . . . People won't do it. But for the tutor it becomes a threatening thing to say: 'Look, you haven't learned enough,' because it means, 'Maybe I haven't been a good enough tutor,' instead of, 'I set a test, you flunked it, it's too bad. . . . You have to do more work.' And students are reluctant to say of one another, 'This person should be held back' although we might say it plenty (privately) and think it plenty. When it really comes right down to saying it in front of the tutor, everybody says, 'Well, it was pretty hard to know what so and so knew.' And you kind of hedge. You never really know. I guess it's a hard thing to evaluate someone's knowledge (Interview: Spring, third year).

Occasionally, an unintended consequence of the "gentleman's agreement" is that students develop a false sense of confidence (or apprehension) because they rely on what they later perceive as less-than-candid assessments by peers and faculty members. Two students comment about this situation in retrospect:

> You always compared yourself with peers and that didn't always work. I tended to take people very literally when they said, 'It's all right, you're doing O.K., take it easy'. . . . I think I'm paying for it now (Interview: Winter, third year).

> It's all you get at this place is that you're doing fine, you're doing all right, everything is going fine. That's the problem. Like we don't know what the expectations are and we don't know what the standards are. Everybody is doing fine, everybody is moving along normally. I wish someone would stand up once in a while, a tutor or whoever, and say: 'Look, this is where you need some work, this is where you're weak, this is the problem for you.' We don't get much of that. What we get are pats on the back (Interview: Winter, third year).

A related worry concerns the effectiveness of evaluations in preparing students to assume the necessary responsibilities that their profession demands. Two students' comments summarize this concern:

I wondered how valid they (evaluations) are. Are we just saying things and they don't really mean anything? We're just gòing through and saying, 'Everything's fine and you're okay and we're all okay'. And I thought, 'Does he, the tutor, know how little I know?' (Interview: Spring, third year).

The difficulty in evaluation comes up in that too often there's glossing over any of the negative or corrective things and too much positive coming out in the evaluation. . . . If there was a lack anywhere, there was a lack of getting realistic, factually based, negative criticism (Interview: Spring, third year).

Another worry expressed about evaluation is specifically related to its interactional nature. Since the students must rely on each other as a source of comparison and evaluation, each must simultaneously avoid being perceived as a threat by other students, gain the approval of both peers and superiors, and attempt to distinguish himself/herself with tutors and clinical preceptors.[4] The result is a subtle competitiveness based on interactional competencies. Two graduating students describe the importance of this kind of skill:

There is always a lot of peer comparison in your tutorials, but oftentimes there are so many other factors involved besides your knowledge . . . like some people are just very verbal. Some people are very aggressive (Interview: Spring, second year).

Evaluation depends partly on what you know. But it really depends on how good a performer you are. . . . In this system that's always true because the tutorial is a verbal system and performers always tend to do well in that anyway (Interview: Spring, second year).

Although the social control of face-to-face evaluation is subtle, it is also powerful. Students taking tests can choose to distance themselves from other participants, but an evaluation system based on the interaction of tutors and peers, demands participation and cooperation. The required self-exposure generally produces anxiety, especially early in the program, which affects interactional skills. Two students make this point:

The biggest difference for me here is that you have to reveal more of yourself. You can't hide yourself. You're open to scrutiny and you expose yourself in the tutorial as part of your education (Field notes: Winter, third year).

In other programs the students are able to be anonymous and sit in class and say nothing. They don't have to reveal much of themselves. We are constantly subject to the scrutiny of others and constantly engaged in addressing others who are evaluating us (Interview: Winter, third year).

The context of interactional evaluation combined with the absence of formal examinations and a grading system breeds uncertainty. As Shibutani (1966) notes happens in many such situations, rumor and gossip are common. When reputations are created and defined in interactional settings, students are concerned about becoming objects displayed for discussion:

But here, I mean, you fart and the next day or later that afternoon everybody in the class knows what is going on. Like so and so does so well, and so and so is having problems. And so and so here is really doing great, he is in the library all the time, and he knows all the answers to the questions.... The gossip is unbelievable (Interview: Spring, second year).

Collectively and individually, then, the students perceive that impression management is critical to convincing evaluators or gatekeepers of their competent trustworthiness:

(In clerkship) how does one person get a good evaluation and another person doesn't. We made this analogy between feathers and black eyes.... If you began in the beginning with too many black eyes, you could never get rid of a black eye. A blue and black eye would always stay there and they would always recognize you with the black eye. It didn't matter how many feathers you got afterwards.... Whereas, if you started off with feathers and you got enough feathers in the beginning, so you almost had a full hatband of feathers, it doesn't matter what you did. One may fall off every now and then.... And then you'd get to a stage where you'd have all these feathers, shit, a whole roll of feathers, and you couldn't for the life of you, you just couldn't get a black eye. You were invincible. You were the big chief. And that's what clerkship is all about—impressing. And if you impress a person enough, and you impress him at a critical time, then that was it—you got your good evaluation (Interview: Spring, third year).

The increased measure of responsibility that comes with

clerkship is accompanied by a broader and more intense scrutiny of the student's clinical capabilities. Their descriptions of clerkship experiences highlight the diversity of their audiences and the variability of expectations:

> Clerkship, it's difficult because you're under scrutiny all the time. I'm particularly anxious about the staff because they have such conflicting ideas about medicine. You see the thing that we find out is that medicine is not so much a science—it's really much more of an art (Field notes: Fall, third year).

Frequent changes of assignment and the nature of hospital organization combine to ensure a high turnover of audiences for the clerk. There is often considerable ambiguity about which script is appropriate for a particular audience.

> A lot of types of guys (doctors), like certain obstetricians, like their thing done a certain way. They like their episiotomies done this way, you know. I mean they like them (women) sewn up in a particular way. You know, there is a certain way to do it, and this is the right way, my way. If you're going to deliver one of my babies, then you've got to do it my way or else you don't do it (Interview: Winter, third year).

The entire situation is clearly an initiation or ritual ordeal (Lortie, 1968; Haas et al., 1982). A student summarizes the sense of self-exposure, mortification, and insufficiency:

> It's whole new ball game when you become a clerk. All of a sudden you're the easy fool. Nurses are laughing at you, doctors are ordering you around, telling you how stupid you are and how you never learned anything. All of a sudden you've got to deal with all these things and you don't have the protection of the library and the cafeteria that you had before. . . . You've got to figure out how to survive in a situation where you don't know a whole lot, but you're expected to know more than you do (Interview: Fall, third year).

As this speaker suggests, the clerk's critics and legitimators are not restricted to persons who are officially responsible for reviewing and appraising performances. Supporting actors and even bit players in the hospital drama are also important:

> In order to do those things (perform competently in clerkship), number one, the biggest thing for that is to really know how to get along with

people—the people you have to work with. And if you don't hit it off right with the nurses, it's over, it's over. You've had it and you might as well pack it up (Field notes: Spring, third year).

Because nurses and other ancillary medical personnel are involved in situations in which the clerk is required to perform competently, they often provide the most immediate feedback about successful execution of the role:

> You are on the ward, the nurses are saying, 'Hey, you've got this patient going down the tube.' You are it. And what do you do . . . ? Now, when you can handle situations like that, you find you are competent. The nurses will see that, and they will say, 'Gee, that was damn good. Gee, that guy really knows his stuff and he handled that fantastic' (Field notes: Spring, second year).

The use of impression-management skills is less critical with patients with whom the student has to exercise little responsibility. Patients are, however, potential critics of student performances. A student points out their "crap-detecting" (Postman and Weingartner, 1969) potential when she says:

> When people are trying to bullshit the patients you could just see the look on the patient's face when they were explaining things, and the patient knew, 'Well, that's a bunch of horse shit' because you'd done it on them three times before. . . . So far it's worked out better being honest with the patients saying, 'Well I've got a couple of ideas but nothing sort of fits right and at my stage of the game I want to try. . . . (Field Notes: Spring, second year.)

The fragility of students' control over others' impressions is exacerbated because some perceive their initiation as being, at times, malicious. Two students observe:

> Part of the sadistic fun of consultants are the ways that consultants amuse themselves by confronting students with things they are undoubtedly not going to know. Like, 'What is the so and so murmur and what is the so and so murmer?' Well first of all, it might not even be in the book and they have heard about it on the round once when someone humiliated them . . . . That is the way life is in this business and some people get kicks, they get sadistic kicks out of this sort of thing (Interview: Winter, third year).

Right now they are getting their shots at us. One way that you can think of clerkship is that it is a stepping stone for somebody else's ego. Everybody gets to pick on you (Field notes: Fall, third year).

## THE SITUATION OF McMASTER STUDENTS

It has already been noted that in early clinical experiences all medical students face varying expectations from a variety of legitimators, some of which are quite cynical in their dealings with students. Students deal with changing expectations from legitimators by carefully managing the image they project. It is true that the nontraditional program at McMaster makes self impression-management more crucial, but, at the same time, it does provide students with some excellent opportunities to develop this skill.

It can happen that in the hospitals used for the school's clerkships, the students are supervised and evaluated by practitioners who may be unenthusiastic about the McMaster approach. One area of contention concerns the school's lack of emphasis on acquiring a core of biomedical facts. A student says:

The problems are people accepting you as a Mac student . . . . A lot of people know McMaster students are weak in their anatomy so they say something like, 'What nerve goes to this and this and this? Oh, you wouldn't know, you're a Mac student' (Field notes: Spring, third year).

Another student offers:

They [cynics about the innovative approach] are looking for our weakness. And you get very angry with the surgeon who keeps on picking at you about anatomy when he knows you haven't studied it. You know they are purposely trying to make you feel insecure. They are doing it on purpose (Field notes: Fall, third year).

Students also find that McMaster's pedagogical emphases on problem-solving and the psychosocial aspects of medicine are sometimes irrelevant to the demands of clerkship. A student summarizes the conflict existing between McMaster's innovative program and the demands of a traditional faculty:

The problem-based approach is a myth when you get into clerkship. You can't take your patient and then disappear to the library conveniently and do over the various differential diagnoses, mainly because the clerkship program is run primarily by people who haven't been trained at Mac . . . . In fact, I had a classical interaction with one of the people I was working with. . . . I was supposed to review a couple of patients with him and he stopped me cold and he said, 'Don't give me that Mac problem-solving bullshit' (Interview: Spring, third year).

Thus, the students find that their inculcated approach makes some of their audiences 'hard to play to' and does not provide them with all the information others expect them to have.

## ADAPTATIONS FOR THE LICENSING EXAMINATION

In Canada, graduates of any medical education program must pass a national licensing-board examination in order to be certified. Thus as the McMaster student approaches graduation, the licensing examination becomes a source of increasing anxiety and uncertainty. Realizing that the examination is not designed to test new pedagogical approaches and theories, most students become doubtful about the effectiveness of their school's educational methods.

The school gives them no preparation for the examination other than building into the program a six-week period during which no activities are scheduled and that permits students to organize a review phase. Individually and collectively, they resort to traditional techniques for learning, identifying, and memorizing material, techniques which they became familiar with and found useful during earlier pre-medical learning situations. A student preparing for the examination describes the change in approach:

The five weeks that you have for the LMCC' (Licentiate of the Medical College of Canada) is a time when you say, 'Look, this is when I have to throw everything else out and learn stuff which I think is going to be on the LMCC (Interview: Spring, third year).

As classes in previous years had done, the group we observed organized a program of lectures and practice examinations.

These were well-attended. Students anxiously awaited the results of the latter, which were similar in format to the licensing examination, and students developed competency reputations by comparing their "grades" (Bucher and Stelling, 1977; Olesen and Whittaker, 1968). Student organizers even went to the length of posting another medical school's schedule of review lectures. A car-pool was set-up to allow students to get to these lectures; the medical school was an hour's drive away. Students not only attended these lectures, but organized their time to attend yet another two lectures given at McMaster.

The students recognize the contradiction between their methods of studying for the licensing examination and the school's philosophy of problem-solving and self-directed learning, a philosophy they presumably accept. One student says:

> Phase V is basically a cram course. . . . My own feeling about this is that it is just to relieve anxiety. . . . I think it is a bit of a kick in the face from the school's theory. . . . A lot of people . . . . feel this is the place where they are going to learn the things they missed (Interview: Spring, third year).

Many students rationalize their realization of contradictory approaches by claiming their actions are necessary to meet outsiders' expectations. As one student phrases it:

> (Phase V) is the exact opposite of the school's philosophy, to have lectures and to take tests. They [organizers and lecturers] are just trying to get us through the exams (Interview: Spring, third year).

Two students and an observer discuss how perceptions of traditional expectations result in compromises that conflict with the innovative philosophy:

> Observer says, 'I hear that the exam answers in the library have been circled. It sounds to me like the end of problem-solving at McMaster.'
> Tom says: 'That's right. It's a different situation now. We have got to absorb a lot of information preparing for the exam. It doesn't very much allow for the problem-solving approach.'
> Ruth says: 'That happens on the wards as well. It often becomes a patterned recognition thing. . . .'
> Tom replies: 'Yes, you only utilize the problem-solving approach when you have a problem. If you recognize it through patterned recognition, that's fine too' (Interview: Spring, third year).

In other words, the students' uncertainty about successfully meeting professionalizing expectations leads them to organize their behavior in accordance with the mode of evaluation, even though they have adapted to a very different system.

Two aspects of the McMaster curriculum, however, prove beneficial as the students take on the role of clerk. The one is the practice they have had in interactional and impression-management skills; the other is their familiarity with medicine's symbolic props and language. Students in traditional examination based situations learn how to pass examinations by determining and studying those things they are likely to be questioned on (Becker et al., 1961). Students in a group interactional evaluation setting learn to pass those tests which emphasize matters of presentation, tact, and poise. McMaster clerks survive two years in which they meet required standards by handling themselves in group settings, where they manage to strike the right balance between questioning and answering and by drawing attention— but not too much attention—to themselves. In short they effectively utilize the skills they learn in impression management. As one student says of behavior in tutorials:

> You have to say things emphatically. What you want to be able to do is to speak correctly using the right language and forcefully. If you do that, you've got it made. . . . If you are able to talk that way it usually means that you know your business, because it's hard to talk that way. . . . But the most important thing for a medical student to learn is to learn to be emphatic. To act confidently. To act surely (Interview: Winter, third year).

In addition to having had this intensive practice in presenting themselves, McMaster students enter clerkship with the advantage of having had considerable experience with the costumes and props of their profession.

## THE SYMBOLS OF PROFESSIONALISM

The professionalization of medical students is facilitated and intensified by symbols the neophytes manipulate. The manipulation serves to announce to insiders and outsiders alike how they are to be identified. During the first weeks of their studies students begin wearing white lab jackets with plastic name tags which identify them as medical students. In addition, since from the beginning clinical skills sessions are included in the curriculum, students participate in a variety of settings with the tools of the doctor's trade carried on their person. This attire clearly identifies students to participants and visitors of the hospital/school setting. Then, equipped with their identity kit, students begin to learn and express themselves in the medical vernacular, often referred to as "McBabble" or "medspeak." Distinctive dress, badges, tools and language provide the student with symbols which announce their role and activity.

The significance of these symbols to the professionalization process is critical. The symbols serve, on the one hand, to identify and unite the bearers as members of a community of shared interests, purpose and identification (Roth, 1957), and on the other these symbols distinguish and separate their possessors from lay people, making their role seem more mysterious, shrouded, and priest-like (Bramson, 1973). The early manipulation of these symbols serves to heighten identification and commitment to the profession, while at the same time facilitates students' separation from the lay world. As one student candidly remarks:

> Wearing the jacket seems to give you carte blanche to just about go anywhere you want in the hospital. People assume that you belong and that you know what you're doing (Field notes: Spring, second year).

The importance of the white coat as a symbol is reinforced by the faculty and staff who, with the exception of the psychiatry department, mandate that it be worn. As the following incident illustrates, this expectation is rigorously adhered to, and is justified in terms of patients' expectations:

> The rheumatology session tutorial group assembled and walked to the room where Dr. Gordon would be met. Dr. Gordon said, 'Well you know in order to see any of the patients you have to wear a white jacket and a tie.' The group was very surprised by his remark and, in fact, John and Ken looked at each other in disbelief. John said, 'No, I didn't know that.'
> Dr. Gordon says, 'Well you do know that in order to see any of the

patients you have to wear a white coat. They expect that. You will agree that they expect that. Wouldn't you agree with that?'
John says, 'No, I wouldn't. I mean that hasn't been my experience.'
Dr. Gordon says, 'Well, have you ever visited any of the patients in the hospital?'
John says, 'Yes for about a year and a half now.'
Dr. Gordon says, 'Those people who have the white jackets on will be able to visit the patients. Those who don't, won't be able to.' (Field notes: Winter, second year).

One of the first difficult tasks that faces students is to begin to learn and communicate within the symbolic system that serves to define medical work and workers. Learning to use the "correct" language is part of this. From the beginning, in tutorials, readings, demonstrations, and rounds, students are exposed to a language in which they are expected to become facile. A student explains the importance of replacing his lay vocabulary:

When I was just beginning, I would use my own words to describe how a lesion looked or how a patient felt. . . because they were more immediate to me and more accessible to me. And on many occasions I was corrected. The way you describe that is such and such because that is the vocabulary of the profession and that is the only way you can be understood (Interview: Winter, third year).

Another incident that took place in a tutorial captures the students' difficulties in knowing when use of the symbol system may be inappropriate:

At one point Dr. Smith asked, 'What is it, what is the name for this kind of phenomenon that gives this kind of pain?' E.G. volunteered a term and she ended it with a question mark. She was tentatively offering a term. Dr. Smith said, 'Just use the plain language, what is the plain everyday word for that?' There was a pause and he said, 'Heartburn, that's what everybody calls it and that's good enough' (Field notes: Spring, first year).

The separation between "we" and "they" becomes clearer to the students as they learn the professional symbol system and are absorbed into the medical culture. As they move through the culture, they learn how symbols are used to communicate and enforce certain definitions of the situations they are exposed to. Students must learn how practicing physicians manipulate these symbols to this end.

The ability to use the linguistic symbols of medicine defines members of the profession and creates a boundary that is not often crossed. Two students reflect on the significance of technical terminology:

> . . . so you could talk about things in front of a patient that would totally baffle the patient and keep him unaware of issues that you were discussing. I don't think this is unique to medicine. I think this is a general phenomenon of professionalization. [Learning the language] was a matter of establishing some common ground with people you were going to be relating to on a professional basis for the rest of your life (Interview: Spring, third year).

> . . . you just can't survive if you don't learn the jargon. It's not so much an effort to identify as it is an effort to survive. People in medicine have a world unto themselves and a language unto themselves. It's a world with a vocabulary . . . and a vocabulary that, no question about it, creates a fraternity that excludes the rest of the world and it's a real tyranny to lay persons who don't understand it . . . . (Interview: Spring, third year).

In sum, the adoption of special props, costume and language reinforces the students' identification with, and commitment to medicine while it enables them to project an image of having adopted a new and special role. Having learned how to manipulate the symbols to reflect audiences' expectations, they begin to shape and control their professional relationships.

The manipulation of symbolic language and props does more than shape and control professional relationships, it actually changes the neophyte's own perception of himself. Because students wear and manipulate the symbols of their trade, they are presumed by others to possess special knowledge. Not only this, but students, because of a developing facility to manipulate symbols, eventually convince themselves that indeed they are special. One student thoughtfully comments on the dynamic nature of the relationship existing between the symbol system and his own self-image:

> When you wore the jacket, especially in the beginning, people were impressed. After all, it told everyone, including yourself, that you were

studying to be a *doctor*. . . . The other thing about wearing the white jacket is that it does make things more obvious. You know what you are, what you are doing sort of thing. You know, it is sort of another way of identifying. There were very few ways that people had to identify with the medical profession and one of the ways was to begin to look like some of the doctors (Interview: Spring, second year).

## MANAGING THE SITUATION

It must be noted, however, that while appropriate medical accoutrements help new clerks manage their new roles, they remain acutely aware of their limitations, and are highly sensitive to a perceived need that they must meet a variety of role expectations. Their short-term goal is to convince their audience of their competence without inviting criticism: they must gain the confidence of those who can affect their reputation. One student discussed the importance of impression management in relation to varying audience expectations in these terms:

> The first day you've got to make a good impression. If you make a bad impression the first day, then that's it. You've got to spend the whole rest of the rotation redeeming yourself for making a boo-boo. Maybe it's just an insignificant thing, but if you do that the first day, then you've had it (Field notes: Fall, second year).

In their attempt to control their audiences' impressions of them, students usually use two broadly based but intricately related strategies: the first is covering up, a strategy intended to provide protection from charges of incompetence; the second is the necessity of taking initiative. Both strategies are designed to convince others that they are developing the necessary attribute of trustworthy competence. Both strategies require considerable skills in self-presentation. A student describes one the these strategies as a form of initiative taking that provides protection from divergent medical approaches taken by senior personnel:

> Like Dr. Jones who was my advisor or boss for medicine, he always came and did rounds on Tuesday mornings . . . . His interest was in endocrinology and . . . he was going to pick up that endocrine patient to talk about, and so of course Monday night any dummy can read up

Monday night like hell on the new American Diabetic Association standards for diabetes or hyperglycemia. . . . So the next day you seem
fairly knowledgeable. . . . But I just wonder how much you remember
when you try to read over in a hurry and you try to be keen just for the
next day. Because that afternoon you forget about it because you figure
Wednesday morning hematology people make their rounds and, of
course, you have to read hematology Tuesday night (Interview: Winter,
second year).

The constant need to create and manage the image of a
competent self through the process of impression management
is sometimes at odds with a basic tenet of the school's philosophy
that encourages learning through problem-solving, and the
complementary development of a questioning attitude. In order
to deal with this contradiction students attempt to manage an
appearance of competence while at the same time they control
others' impressions of it. This student expresses his handling of
the problem this way:

The best way of impressing others with your competence is asking
questions you know the answers to. Because if they ever put it back on
you, 'Well what do you think?' then you tell them what you think and
you'd give a very intelligent answer because you knew it. You didn't ask
to find out information. You ask it to impress people (Interview:
Winter, third year).

The same contradiction gives rise to another strategy that
students employ designed to mask uncertainty and anxiety with
an image of self-confidence. Projection of the right image is
recognized by students as being as important as technical competence. As one student remarks: "We have to be good actors, put
across the image of self-confidence, that you know it all . . . ."
Another student, referring to the importance of creating the
right impression, claims:

It's like any fraternity. You've got to know. You've got to have a certain
amount of basic knowledge before they think it's worth talking to you.
If you display less than that basic knowledge their reflexes come into
play and they think this person is an idiot. Let's find out exactly how
much they don't know, rather than building on what you do know.
That's a different maneuver. Being out in the pale, not worth talking to,
or within the pale and well-worth talking to. There is image management in every profession. It's very unfortunate because the people who

precisely need the help are those who are willing to admit their ignorance, and I've been in tutorials where people who are really willing to admit their ignorance tend to get put down for it. After a while they stop asking questions. That's very unfortunate (Interview: Spring, third year).

Clinical clerks believe that they must always be aware of the expectations of their audience before they carefully balance a self-confident demeanor with an attitude and gestures of proper deference in the face of those who control their career:

> Student A: Sometimes there is a lot of politics involved . . . in speaking up because you are aware of your position. . . . You don't want to seem too smart. You don't want to show up people. If you happen to know something, you know, that say the resident doesn't know, you have to be very diplomatic about it because some of these guys are very touchy.
> Student B: And you don't want to play the game either of just 'I'll be student and you be teacher'.
> Student A: Yeah, and at the same time you don't want to come off as appearing stupid. If you happen to believe something . . . you try to defend yourself but in a very diplomatic manner, all the time being careful not to step on anybody's toes (Interview: Spring, third year).

The use of presentational skills can only be understood in terms of students' perceptions that impression management offers the most appropriate tactics for successfully negotiating the evaluation system they face (Becker et al., 1961; 1967). Most are quite frank about the importance of consciously impressing others. Two students comment:

> In that context [with the clinical skills preceptor] try to shine. I try to outdo others. It's also good if you raise your hand and give a side-point. . . . You guess with confidence. If you don't know, no matter what, you say it with confidence. You'll be much better on rounds if you do that. . . . (Interview: Spring, second year).

> If you want to establish a reputation as a great staff man or whatever, one of the things is that you know a lot and this is one of the ways you establish your reputation. . . . Some people will cover up by bull-shitting very skillfully. People usually don't make the effort to prove them wrong. And it always helps to be ready with a quick snappy answer which is right. . . . And what I usually do is I say I don't know, but I usually say it with a very aggressive air, you know, but not in a put-down way (Interview: Fall, third year).

The relationship between verbal or interactional skills and reputation-making is highlighted during these student interviews:

> Well, I know people who came across as knowing a lot and they don't do it purposely or they don't do it arrogantly or anything, they just talk a lot. And usually most of these people do know a lot and they talk a lot. But a fair amount of it is also they are just good talkers. They are good with words and if you were to sort of compare them with someone who is less flashier in a different setting, in other words, ask them to do a write-up or ask them to do a written assessment of the patient. The quieter one would probably do just as well. These people are better on their feet so they come across all right. There is definitely that aspect and you see that even more when you get into clinical medicine and really much of what gives a person a reputation is not really how much he knows, although he's got to know a fair amount, he's got to know certainly above average, but really how much of a performer he is (Interview: Spring, third year).

> The way reputations are established on a ward, be it for clinical clerks, interns, residents, or staff is largely on the basis of verbal discussions that occur all over the place. They occur at rounds . . . they occur at seminars and so on. And these are all verbal, that's the big thing about them. At these sorts of goings on, it's people who were quick, who jumped in with a diagnosis when only two symptoms were known and were right, who are good with words and that sort of thing—these sort of people are the ones who tend to establish reputations. Rarely are reputations made on the basis of reading written products of their work. Residents, they do write things. You know, they write discharge summaries, they write admitting histories and physicals. And often times, especially if the patient comes back, these things will be read by another person. In that sense you may get an idea of what the person has done at a quieter time when he hasn't had to perform verbally. By and large, that's a lesser aspect of it than what happens at these sessions. It's really the people who are verbal and sort of aggressive in that way who are known as being good. (Interview: Spring, third year).

Even as they pursue good evaluations through good interactional performances, the students do not ignore their long-term goal of achieving competence. One aptly sums up the relationship of meeting the expectations of frequently changing audiences, and the necessity of impression management, with a lesser but, nonetheless, important concern about his future role as a decision maker.

This week I was at all different places, some of which I had never been to. You're having a constant turnover of patients and a constant turn-over of staff people that you run into. Each of them has different expectations towards you, and you're always on guard. You're never exactly sure how each of them wants you to act, so it puts you in a kind of tension situation. I know when I leave work I really feel a big relief that I can finally let my hair down. Most of us present this image that we are comfortable and confident. That's the image you have to present. . . . I figure to myself as a doctor you shouldn't have to feel this way, but I think one thing medical school does to you is by the time you graduate you realize how little you do know and how much there is to know. And it's so overwhelming to see your finiteness and limitations, and to recognize when you get the degree, all of a sudden you're going to be expected to know. You're going to be expected to make decisions (Interview: Winter, third year).

## Performance Success and Professionalizing Confidence and Identification

As they advance through the program, students continually observe doctors' working habits, listen to their philosophies of medical practice, take note of their competencies and incompetencies, and reflect upon the nature of their own present and future relationships with patients. The physicians with whom they practice their clinical skills become models after which students pattern their own beliefs and behavior:

> . . . certainly there are people who impress me . . . certain aspects of their personality that I would want to incorporate in some way in my practice. It is easy to model yourself after people you see on the wards. . . . You don't know anything and you start watching them and before too long you find yourself in a position where you tend to model yourself after these people. . . .

Through observation, role-playing, and practice, students begin to identify with the organization and practice of the medical profession.

As students observe and experience the problems of medical care and practice, they develop an understanding of, and learn to identify with, the profession and the means by which its members confront their problems. Consequently, students became less able to voice criticisms of what they see as they adopt the role of those they will emulate in the future. As they assume increased responsibilities and make medical judgments for which they must account to a variety of professionals, they develop an increasingly sympathetic outlook towards their future profession.

Students gain clinical and interactional experience in ward settings that allows them to increase their repertoire of roles played for various audiences and in different situations. A student describes her experiments with various scripts when she says:

> Every patient I see gives me more experience. I'll see as many patients as I can because I can learn from seeing them. Like I can try out a different approach and see the reaction that I get. I found that every time I see a patient, I try to ask questions in a different way and test out different approaches. It's like going to see a play that you've already seen many times, but every time you see it you notice something different. In a sense it's the same with the patients. You gain a little more experience every time, and that is really important (Interview: Spring, second year).

It would appear that nothing succeeds like success; and as the students gain confidence they learn that the projection of a successful image is an effective way of controlling others' impressions of their developing professionalism. A student describes the importance of impression-management skills in easing their relationships with patients, particularly in dealing with the sensitive areas of the physical examination:

> I think it's largely a matter of how you present yourself. Now if I go in all shaky and flushed and nervous about it, the patient is going to pick up on this and is going to respond. So I think you have to go in with a confident manner and know your business and go about it in a very clear cut way, so the patient does not know you have any fears of the situation and therefore you don't transfer those fears to the patient (Interview: Winter, third year).

Another student graphically describes the ambiguous nature of interactional evaluation and the skills required to handle the ambiguity. Students believe they can deflect others from evaluating cognitive or performance competence negatively.

You see the kind of student that they [faculty] want to see is the strong and the assertive-type person. Medical people like to see people who state their position and take a stand . . . a go-getter, an individual who can relate, an individual who on their own can lead a tutorial group, who can take patients and follow them through, who can take initiatives. . . . If they see you being decisive and confident and they see you can do something, then they think you're good. I think it's very easy for you to slide by on personality. Sometimes I think I'm at fault . . . because I think I have the personality that I can put others in the situation where they won't go and find out if I'm weak in some areas. That's the problem with this place: that they never really separate personality from academics (Interview: Winter, second year).

As students gain confidence they learn that skillful methods of communication provides an effective way of controlling others' impressions of their professionalism. The intimate relationship between developing confidence and professional success through the projection of confident performances that convey success is indicated in the following student's comments:

If you act like you know, they treat you like you know. If you act like you don't know what is happening, then that's the way they treat you. It might sound really strange, but that is the way it is. You've got to let them know that you know what you are doing (Field notes: Fall, third year).

Confidence is often bolstered by the comparisons that students inevitably make with their peers and practicing professionals; the clerks realize that other players too, are involved in the game of impression management. Lack of knowledge and even incompetence are easy to hide in a milieu that emphasizes appearance.[5] A student makes this point:

The comforting thing about clerkship is that you see that specialists and interns and residents don't know everything. That's kind of reassuring to know that first of all you don't have to know everything and secondly that a lot of people who are beyond you in their training don't know everything (Field notes: Spring, third year).

Clerks are in continuous contact with other members of the medical hierarchy and thus have ample opportunity to imitate them. Conforming to the model of their evaluators makes them aware that professional practice is a mixture of both science and art. The art of impression management when mastered allows the clerks to increase their identification with the practice, and allows them to gain confidence about their ability to demonstrate professional competence. Eventually, successful completion of the clerkship provides a social badge of legitimation, which affirms they have taken another step in the transition from student to professional.

In summary, the students come to realize that as practicing professionals, they will continue to place emphasis on the symbolic communication of competence. Effective reputation-making, for practitioners as well as for students, depends on the successful control and manipulation of symbols, ideas, and legitimators in professional rituals and situations. Donald Light astutely points out the outcome of what amounts to a ritual ordeal in the study of psychiatric residents when he notes:

> By structuring them (training programs) so that the trainees experience feelings of intense anxiety, ignorance, and dependence, such programs may be teaching professionals to treat clients as they have been treated. And by exaggerating their power and expertise, mentors establish a model of omnipotence that their students are fated to repeat. To the extent that laymen accept this mythology, omnipotent tendencies become reinforced in daily life. To the extent they challenge it, professionals like physicians or psychiatrists become embattled and defensive (1980:307).

A key factor in the professionalization process is that students learn authoritativeness is communicated by means of body language, demeanor, and carefully managed projections of the self-image. They believe that to be a good student-physician is either to be or appear to be competent. They observe that others react to their role playing. A student describes this process when he says:

> To be a good GP, you've got to be a good actor, you've got to respond to a situation. You have to be quick, pick up the dynamics of what is going on at the time and try to make the person leave the office thinking that you know something. And a lot of people, the way they handle that is by letting the patient know that they know it all and only letting out a little bit at a time, and as little as possible. I think that they eventually reach a plateau where they start thinking to themselves they are really great

and they know it all, because they have these people who are worshipping at their feet (Interview: Spring, third year).

The self-fulfilling nature of the conversion process, whereby newcomers attain the higher moral status of a professional, is captured in two separate interview comments:

People expect you to be the healer and so you have to act like the healer. (Field notes: Spring, third year.)

You know a large part of our role is a God role. You have to act like God. You're supposed to be like God. If you don't inspire confidence in your patients, they are not going to get better even if you know the correct diagnosis and have the correct treatment. If they don't have faith in you, they are not going to get better (Interview: Winter, second year).

The perception of exaggerated expectations from their audience and the ritual ordeal nature of the professionalization process contribute to the model of omnipotence that students believe is helpful for performance success. There is, however, a fine line and tension between confident acting and audience perceptions of arrogance and abuse of authority. The root of this dilemma is reflected in Lord Acton's famous dictum, 'Power tends to corrupt and absolute power tends to corrupt absolutely.' A clinical clerk describes the corruptive tendency of the professionalizing process when he says:

They [the nurses] expect you to act that way [abusively]. If you don't, they won't respect you. They need to know you're the boss or they won't respect you (Field notes: Spring, third year).

The process of adopting the cloak of competence is ultimately justified by students as being helpful to the patient. A student summarizes the relationship between acting competently and patients responding to such a performance by getting well when he says:

You know the patients put pressure on you to act as if you are in the know. If you know anything about the placebo effect, you know that a lot of the healing and curing of patients does not involve doing anything that will really help them, but rather creating confidence in the patient that things are being done and will be done. We know that the placebo effect for example has even cured cancer patients. If they have the confidence in the doctor and what doctor and what treatment they are undergoing, they are much more likely to get well, irrespective of the objective effects of the treatment (Interview: Spring, second year).

## CONCLUSION

Students learn the practical importance of assuming the cloak of competence.[6] The cloak allows patients to trust, without question, both the health professional and the prescribed treatment. Successful negotiations of the trial by ordeal through proper performances helps newcomers gain control or dominance (Friedson, 1970) which is basic to professionalism. The process has a self-fulfilling quality as neophyte professionals move up the professional ladder. Students recognize the importance of appearing authoritative in professional situations. In turn, as they perceive themselves to be successful, they come to believe in their competence in professional matters. The changing nature of the definition of self and the fragility of control over others' perceptions and reactions leads students to develop and maintain a protective shield.

The posture of authoritativeness in professional matters is an expected outcome of the trial by ordeal. The special status and role of professional is enveloped in a set of expectations that require special demonstrations of "possessed" competence. Practicing at playing the role eventually results in its adoption and identification. Newcomers model and imitate their mentors (who are also responsible for evaluating them) and the self-perpetuation of the notion of their having a special authoritativeness proceeds.

Neophytes and professionals are similarly involved in careers based on reputational control. Indeed, many laypeople are not only aware that the professionals they deal with are almost constantly engaged in playing a part, in projecting the 'proper' image, they demand it. The interactional basis for this adaptation to a lifetime role is summarized by Halmos when he says:

We must conclude that the role-playing of being a professional is a hard social fact, and a potent behavioural model for the nonprofessionals, and thus for society at large. . . . The strange thing is that the world cannot afford to dispense with being systematically conned! Of course, the truth is that the world is not being deceived: it demands the professing of values and their embodiment in a culturally defined style and ritual (1970:180–181).

In his study of the mentally retarded, Edgerton (1967) maintains that the central and shared commonality of the mentally retarded released from institutions was for them to envelop themselves in a cloak of competence to deny the discomforting reality of their stigma. The development of a cloak of competence is, perhaps, most apparent for those who must meet exaggerated expectations. The problem of meeting others enlarged expectations is magnified for those uncertain about their ability to manage a convincing performance. Moreover, the performer faces the personal problem of reconciling his provate self-awareness and uncertainty with his publicly displayed image. For those required to perform beyond their capacities, in order to be successful, there is the constant threat of breakdown or exposure. For both retardates and professionals the problem and, ironically, the solution, are similar. Expectations of competence are dealt with by strategies of impression management, specifically, manipulation and concealment. Interactional competencies depend on convincing presentations and much of professionalism requires the masking of insecurity and incompetence with the symbolic-interactional cloak of competence.

As Hughes has observed, ". . . a feature of work behavior found in one occupation, even a minor or odd one, will be found in others" (1952:425). In fact, the basic processes of social life operate throughout the social structure. All social groups create boundaries and differences, view themselves in the most favorable ways.[7] All individuals and groups strive to protect themselves from ridicule and charges of incompetence. Our analysis has captured what is and has been a "taken-for-granted" understanding of social life: much behavior is performance designed to elicit certain reactions. In fact, as we maintain, professional behavior is, or can be, understood as performance.[8]

# Chapter VI

# *The Waning of Idealism*

This chapter traces what happens to the early idealism of student doctors. Our findings show that loss of idealism goes beyond a temporary diversion caused by situational demands of medical school. Rather it is inherent in the very demands of professionalization. We begin by describing students' changing perceptions of the importance of psychosocial issues in medicine. In their need to strive for competence, students 'turn off' their emotional reactions to patients. Equally important is the students' perception of the medical profession's expectation of affective neutrality towards patients. We conclude that loss of idealism must be understood in the context of a symbolic-moral drama wherein professionalization is conceptualized as a process of differentiation and alienation from lay society and of elevation to a position of detachment and control.

In many, perhaps all fields, professionalization entails a radical reorientation to the goals and methods of the work—a shedding of prior, often lofty conceptions of how professionals ought to work—and a concomitant adoption of the ways in which they actually behave and think. The shift is, at the same time, both real and symbolic of the neophytes' conversion to the special status of professionals. The inner and outer change, is particularly apparent among medical students. These students generally enter medical school with high hopes of achieving a humanistic, caring approach to patients. Eventually, they emerge from their classroom and clinical experiences demonstrating both by their actions and words, that they are convinced that pragmatism and a stance of affective neutrality are in both their own and patients' best interests.

We are scarcely the first researchers to note this loss of transformation of idealism among student doctors (Becker and Geer, 1958; Olesen and Whittaker, 1968; Simpson, 1972). In 1958, Howard S. Becker and Blanche Geer, in their now classic article, "The Fate of Idealism in Medical School," described adaptations they had observed students making in response to the professionalizing experience.

Our findings complement and support Becker and Geer's, even though 25 years have passed and we observed students in an innovative program designed to emphasize medicine's psychosocial aspects (in contrast to the traditional schools that emphasize the "hard" medical sciences). We differ, however, in our analysis.

Becker and Geer's central argument is that the students ". . . develop cynical feelings in specific situations directly associated with their medical school experience . . . ." (p. 50). They begin their studies with an idealistic perspective, but a series of immediate concerns requires that they place it in abeyance. Students must digest a vast amount of information in a limited time; they must discover the expectations of the faculty in order to pass examinations; perhaps most significantly, they must meet the sometimes variable expectations of faculty and staff in a wide range of clinical experiences. These demands, suggest Becker and Geer, require many internal and external adaptations; the result is a culture that encourages students to focus ". . . their attention almost completely on their day-to-day activities in school and obscures or sidetracks their earlier idealistic preoccupations" (p. 52).

Contrary to Becker and Geer's findings, we note that the students we studied became reconciled to the profession's ways of doing things and adopted rationales provided by the profession itself. Rather than salvaging their ideals by postponing their application to a future time, they became increasingly convinced that the demands of professionalization, which do not lend themselves to an idealistic approach, are unlikely to change or be successfully challenged. Moreover, our data suggest that students perceived the loss of idealism as inherent in the demands of professionalization; medicine is organized on the assumption that practitioners will maintain a psychological distance from patients, and the profession's gatekeepers, consciously or unconsciously, insist that neophytes assume this posture. Further, our analysis emphasizes the significance of the manipulation of appropriate symbolism in facilitating the students' separation from lay culture and clients.

Thus, we suggest, medical students' initial idealism is soon compromised by both the stringencies of their curriculum, stated and hidden, and the demand that they assume the ideology of the profession. If they are to complete the passage to professionalism, idealistic attitudes must go. Idealism is fated to change even in a program designed to enhance it, where psychosocial approaches are valued. The demands for conformity to a professionalizing perspective of affective neutrality to ensure control over professional situations limits the effects of innovation. Whether traditional or innovative program or graduate, the idea remains that a doctor is a doctor, surrounded by the core expectation that he/she be trusted in serious or fateful matters. Such trust is revealed in performances that demonstrate both inner and outer control of reactions that threaten the ideal of scientific and personal objectivity.

This chapter will trace its fading. We begin by describing students' changing perceptions of the importance of psychosocial issues in medicine. Most enter the program convinced that "good" doctors should emphasize these aspects of health care. Yet as they become concerned about meeting professionalizing expectations, which seem to focus on learning the biomedical paradigm, they come to see psychosocial issues as peripheral to "real" medicine. Similarly, they begin their studies with an idealistic concern for the sick as individual, whole human beings. Yet, first in their need to learn as much as possible, then in their desire to act like their mentors, they discover the necessity of depersonalizing patients by treating them as specimens or objects.

Neither change, (particularly the second) comes easily, but the profession does supply rationales. As students observe the routine nature of patient objectification and learn the collective justifications for it, they are prepared for personal change. The ideological reason for developing affective neutrality is coupled with the taking on and manipulation of professional symbols that ease and support neophytes' loss of idealism, which is part of their moral and psychological transformation into physicians.

## THE WANING OF PSYCHOSOCIAL CONSIDERATIONS

As we noted earlier students enter medical school with a complement of ideas about helping the sick and rendering service to humanity. Their foremost concern is the patient, for whom they believe they share a special and sacred responsibility. Their expressed motives for wanting to study medicine are noble and idealistic. They claim monetary considerations are not important, and most actively resent any suggestion of crass or material motives.[1] The following remarks, offered shortly after the student entered the program, reflect the general idealism about future powers and responsibilities:

> I think a large part of what we should be doing is trying to understand people, if you take the perspective, as I do, that a lot of their problems are caused because of alienation. . . you've got to recognize that people come to see you . . . in a doctor role because you are someone who is powerful and they want to seek your advice and counsel. I think we have a responsibility to try and relate to these people, to understand and communicate with them rather than just prescribe (Interview: Winter, first year).

As this and many other students' statements suggest, the beginners feel that "good" doctors should go well beyond "narrow" considerations of specific health problems and deal with the patient as a whole human being who exists within an environment. In other words, they are committed to the psychosocial aspects of medicine. Many students in fact, entered this medical school rather than a more traditional one, because it has a reputation for emphasizing this aspect of medicine.

In many ways, the early curriculum meets this expectation. Phase I—the first ten weeks—is largely an introduction to psychosocial considerations in health care. Discussion in the tutorial groups typically centers on psychosocial issues. Yet in spite of this emphasis and the students' original, idealistic concerns, we observed their interest in psychosocial matters begin to dim almost as soon as their training began. Towards the end of Phase I students openly complained about the excessive attention to psychosocial issues A student summarizes this general attitude:

> There is a real over-kill and it tends to turn people off . . . just so much that I was close to being turned off on a lot of psychosocial issues (Interview: Fall, first year).

For students with little background in the social sciences, psychosocial concerns were perceived as "just going around in circles." A student with a hard science background reflects this concern:

> . . . I don't know what the stuff is really all about. Like it's so nebulous to me. It's so abstract, that I really don't know how to deal with it (Field notes: Winter, first year).

The most significant reason for students' need to shift their focus from the psychosocial to the more clinical aspects of health care seems to relate both to their idealized perceptions of medicine and to their anticipation of the responsibilities they will soon be expected to meet. Although analytically separate, these concerns merge in shaping the students' reaction to psychosocial concerns. The vast majority of students initially regard medicine as a fairly exact science deeply rooted in biochemistry. In this view, the contribution of the social sciences towards explaining and controlling health and illness can only be tangential. Moreover, the body of medical information is enormous, and the students quickly perceive that there is too much to know and little time in which to learn it (Fox, 1957; Haas et al., 1981). Time becomes a precious commodity that must be spent wisely. Thus, they decide, its most efficient use involves absorbing as much biomedical information as possible. In this context, the psychosocial components of the program interferes with a productive use of time:

> One thing you have to do at medical school is pick up all the pathophysiology and to pick up all of the anatomy and pick up the clinical histories, the presentations, the clinical skills and so on. So psychosocial

time is really a luxury, it can't really be afforded sometimes. . . . Do you want to learn a lot of what we call the core material . . . or do you want to rehash a lot of arguments that are of fundamental human importance but really can't be resolved within a reasonable time limit (Interview: Fall, second year).

More advanced students and faculty members endlessly remind beginners that their time in medical school will pass quickly. Furthermore, from the outset of the program, the students are sensitized to the wide range of responsibilities accompanying the physician role and exposed to the important, sometimes fateful matters over which their advice and decision-making will eventually be crucial. Individually and collectively, they face the anxiety-provoking problem of beginning to develop a trustworthy competence. The usually compulsive striving for an appropriate professional competence is intimately related to the decision to devote themselves almost exclusively to learning biomedicine—and to the fading of initial idealism. Two students observe:

Listen, we've got to know medicine and we've got to be able to decipher the situation, to be able to diagnose successfully and be able to outline a plan of treatment. It's not a matter that we don't care [about the psychosocial], but that we can't really afford to if we are to be competent (Field notes: Winter, second year).

With our individual pressure and pressure around us, I don't feel I had time to do something else. It was so much to get through medicine . . . and no groups wanted to spend time with psychosocial issues and I didn't either (Field notes: Winter, third year).

Most students do, however, continue to believe that psychosocial matters are important. However, they assign this area a much-reduced priority, believing that it must be neglected, at least temporarily, in the interests of acquiring as much medical knowledge and competence as possible. As they move through the program, their concern about these issues waxes and wanes as they respond to specific situational requirements and attempt to demonstrate their developing competence and trustworthiness.

The waning of idealism from the altruism expressed at admissions can be fruitfully understood as part of the performance ritual of professionalization. As students move through the program, they learn that the profession, through its representatives, expect competent appearing performances. Contrary to the ideas expected at admissions, where concern for others is important, students perceive that they are expected to suppress emotional feelings which might reflect an absence or lack of control. They learn instead that the professionalizing expectation requires a posture of detached concern consistent with the profession's claim of affective neutrality. Their personal transformation into a professional role requires a shedding of prior conceptions and performances, and an adoption of the profession's perspective of control over emotive situations and reactions of the self.

### Turning Off Your Feelings

A basic problem for the medical practitioner is emotional control and functioning in the face of life-and-death situations. Given their idealism, neophytes in particular must learn to distance themselves from clients by covering and controlling their emotions. Although students initially express considerable anxiety about achieving this adaptation, they need not search far to recognize a collective solution (Becker et al., 1960): it is provided by the very profession for which they are being trained. Their sense of idealism, they learn, is noble, but their progress through medical school requires objectification of the patient. This is one of the major accommodations they must make to the system of organized medicine.

The accommodation is generally made in two steps. The first is primarily a response to situational demands, and many students regard it as temporary. The second is the true conversion that is demanded of them for the ritual passage to professionalization.

### Objectifying the Patient for Learning Purposes

The primary vehicle for teaching students objectivity is the clinical skills sessions in hospital settings. Early in their program, students encounter striking examples of the way in which the profession subjugates patients' needs, rights, and dignities to the clinical tasks at hand. Initially, students are often dismayed by the way in which physicians and other hospital staff members treat patients:

> What I do remember about Phase II that really got me when I did go to a cancer clinic . . . and I saw the way they were just herding in ladies that had hysterectomies and cancer, and just the way the doctors would walk right in and wouldn't even introduce us as students, and just open them up and just look and say a lot of heavy jargon. And the ladies would be saying, 'How is it?' 'Am I better, or worse?' And they say in this phony reassuring tone, 'Yes, you're fine,' and take you into the hallway and say how bad the person was (Interview: Fall, second year).

In the student cohort we observed, the reaction of outrage was strikingly reflected during Phase I by a protest against what a number interpreted as a violation of patients' rights. Students posted and signed a petition expressing their dissatisfaction with the way in which patients were treated as objects for repeated observation and examination.

More often than not, however, the students are reluctant to challenge their evaluators and legitimators:

> They hardly talked to the patient at all. We'd get in there and he'd hold the speculum and we'd all take a look and we would just herd right out again into another room and have a look and herd out again. I thought the dehumanization was awful. . . . I didn't tell the doctor how I felt at the time, but when I left, other people felt the same way. . . . And we sort of bitched to each other how rough it was and how we were going to do something about it and we never did. We let it slide by (Interview: Spring, second year).

A holistic approach may remain the student's goal, but it is soon replaced in practice by a pedagogical conception of the patient as the presentor of clinical symptoms—a teaching and learning device. As one student says:

> Like at the very beginning we're told that the reason we go see these patients is because they can teach us something. . . . That is the only interest that we have in the patients. We aren't there to try to cheer the patient up or to make things easier for the patient. All we are there for is to learn (Interview: Fall, third year).

Eventually students become committed to the idea that patients are objects—material to learn from. As was noted in the previous chapter they believe this is (at least temporarily) necessary if they are to learn clinical symptoms and pathology. Thus, they are adding to their medical knowledge and competence:

> I think you realize there is a structural problem, and there are a lot of demands made on you and you are forced to act in certain ways just to accomplish your work. But right now in the training phase, I find if the clinical preceptor takes me around to listen to six patients with heart murmurs and I only have five minutes with each patient, I don't get concerned if I'm not getting it on with the patient, because I'm trying to learn about heart murmurs (Interview: Winter, second year).

Students' concerns about learning medicine, making the most efficient use of time, and establishing some bases of certainty and security in their work are all reflected in the selective interests they take in patients with unusual pathology (Becker et al., 1961). Discussing the kind of patients that he looks forward to seeing, a student claims:

> A patient who has physical findings. Gees, I don't care what the findings are. It's a fantastic experience to see that physical finding. . . . Someone can tell you this is the way to feel for a lump in the stomach, but if there is no lump there you are not going to learn how to feel it. . . . I think that's what I get the most out of, getting exposure to the pathology (Field notes: Winter, second year).

The goal for the student becomes knowing with some assurance that his or her diagnosis is valid and the treatment competent. A student hypothesizes about such noteworthy experiences:

> I think the magic moments are when someone goes in to see a patient and they haven't seen their records or charts, and they come up with their own diagnosis. And they get the charts and they've discovered some rare tropical disease that they had and they got it on the head. That's the magical moment I've heard of (Field notes: Spring, second year).

The dominant concern with learning medicine leads students to focus their time and energy on learning efficiently. They soon find that they have no time for the frills of emotional involvement and quickly learn to shut down feelings that interfere with their work (Lief and Fox, 1963) and with immediate productivity. As one student says:

You can't function if you think about things like that . . . [death and dying]. Everything you see sort of gets in there and turns about in your mind and you aren't productive. The reason you have to shut it off is because you won't be productive. . . . I think that my prime objective is to learn the pathology (Interview: Winter, third year).

Thus, striving for competence is the initial professionalizing rationale to explain avoiding or shutting off emotional reactions.

### Assuming a Professional Stance

Soon the students take the next step and come to see detachment as part of the professional situation, the routine way to deal with the situation, an expectation over which they exercise little control. They conclude that if they appear to feel for patients and become involved with them, their legitimators will not see them as learning to become professionally competent:

When you see someone who is going to die, especially when you're still learning, you're really cut off from the personal level. You just clue into the pathology. You really shut off. You sort of turn it out of your mind and this person is going to die. You just look at the pathology. . . . You don't really think, "What about the family? What they must be going through. . . ." You can't fall to pieces because you find your patient is going to die in three months or is rapidly going downhill. You have a role to play here (Interview: Fall, third year).

A critical factor influencing the pace at which students realign their idealism and change their perception of the profession and its practices is the way in which they come to realize that their best interests are served in conforming to the demands and expectations of faculty members—the profession's gatekeepers and control agents. Students catch (sooner or later) the many hints dropped from the outset suggesting that some form of accommodation will be required to reconcile the discrepancy between the idealized and actual realities of medicine:

(The Dean) said when we first came here we would be as idealistic as we would ever be, and we would see many abuses and problems in medicine, but that by the time we graduated we would accommodate ourselves to the system of organized medicine (Field notes: Spring, second year).

. . . there are a lot of us who are interested in the more general social issues when we came here, but they took care of that when they took us on a tour of Stelco [a steel factory] at the very beginning of the program. Now everybody in the community knows that Stelco's pumping out stuff that's killing people, but there is no way you are going to do anything about it. (Field notes: Winter, second year).

Quickly or slowly, reluctantly or otherwise, students learn that they do not have time for both learning and caring, and they must stifle their feelings because of the higher value their legitimators place on a "professional" approach or affective neutrality (Coombs and Powers, 1975; Daniels, 1960; Emerson, 1970; Kadushin, 1962; Parsons, 1951). The following student's views are typical:

Look, as I see it, you can't afford to care too much. You keep your feelings at a distance because we have a phrase for it—we call it being professionally responsible. . . . You can't allow your feelings to interfere (Field notes: Fall, third year).

Gradually the students alter their understanding of how medicine should be practiced. Unable to feel as deeply concerned about the patient's total condition as they once believed they should, they adopt a functionally-specific approach (Parsons, 1951) that justifies concentrating only on the individual medical problem. As a student remarks:

Somebody will say 'Listen to Mrs. Jones' heart. It's just a little thing flubbing on the table.' And you forget about the rest of her. Part of that is the objectivity and it helps in learning in the sense that you can go in to a patient, put your stethoscope on the heart, listen to it and walk out. . . . The advantage is that you can go in a short time and see a patient, get the important thing out of the patient and leave (Interview: Winter, third year).

Students discover that such experiences are a routine feature of the hospital setting, regularly accepted by the medical profession. They heed the reminders that their primary objective at this stage of their careers is to absorb as much pathology as possible. More importantly, however, they learn to accept the rationale that a physician's high case load precludes attending to anything but the patient's medical condition.

As students progress through the program, they become increasingly aware of the belief that emotional feelings are a hindrance, that patients must be objectified and depersonalized or the doctor cannot maintain clinical objectivity (Coombs and Powers, 1975; Emerson, 1970). Most students, like the following speaker, accept the view that personal concerns for the patient should not intrude on the physician's role and responsibility:

> This is a really stupid analogy but it probably rings true too. When you go bowling you can't worry about selling your house. You want a good score, yet you're being a human and still bowling. . . . And it's essentially the same kind of thing you have to deal with at various treatment levels with the patient. If you are talking to the family you've got to bring back all those emotions and you've got to use them. If you are dealing with a nursing staff and deciding how you're going to change the solutions and what type of drug you're going to add to this guy's regimen, you can't be saying: 'Oh the poor bastard, we're going to stick another needle in him.' You can't do that (Interview: Spring, second year).

In due course, the students adopt the profession's rationale that their growing detachment from patients is in the latter's best interests, that patients themselves prefer such a response from the physician. A student expresses this view:

> Now there are really very few people, very few patients who want their doctor to be the one who is going to sit there and cry over them, because really they are looking to get out of this predicament they're in. . . . Most patients would be very uncomfortable if they saw you in that state (Interview: Fall, third year).

For the majority of students, the process of objectifying patients is a natural outcome of striving to demonstrate a developing and maturing competence in a relatively short period of time. However removed this approach may be from the individual's private views of medicine and doctor-patient relationship, it is readily justifiable. Furthermore, the student can take comfort in realizing that she/he is not alone, that the approach is common to others in the class as well.

### Personal Change and Symbolic Supports

The journey to medicine's professional ideology is indeed an ordeal for some students. Since personal feelings cannot be easily cast aside, many attempt to balance the need for empathy vis-à-vis the patient with the perceived expectation of emotional detachment:

> ... you should have some feeling and empathy for your patients, but you can't carry the pain around or you wouldn't be able to function. I mean there's a balancing act that you have to make in order to be able to be a successful doctor. (Field notes: Winter, third year.)
>
> ... you have to be objective enough so that you can see things in a way that they can't or else you're not being therapeutic. So I can see the value of keeping a certain hold on yourself and not completely letting yourself go.... In time when you don't have time, you have to put your feelings aside. But I think that on a day-to-day basis you can be ... a <u>mentch</u> [decent person].... (Interview: Spring, third year).

The matter is not easily resolved. In their more private moments, the students, as if feeling that their changing attitudes and behavior are not fully within their control, express the hope—almost like a prayer—that they will not lose sight of the human dimensions in medicine:

> Well, I for one, hope I'll always keep caring and feeling. I hope that every time I give a patient a shot that I realize the pain that's involved.... I hope I don't stop caring.... I think that's too much of what happens at this place that people stop caring, and they become professionalized and they develop excuses for not being more human (Interview: Spring, second year).

> I hope I don't lose the humanistic parts of me. I can see where it's a problem, one that you have to be sensitive to and be careful about losing. I mean part of what they are trying to do is professionalize us and part of being professional, I guess, is to be less human and more objective (Interview: Winter, second year).

For the majority of students, however, changes in attitude and behavior are gradual, and for some, even imperceptible, noticeable only as they become exposed to settings in which they observe the practice of medicine: For example:

Student: I guess I saw it [medicine] as a way of dealing with people in a positive way, in a way that I could help them sort their problems. . . .

Observer: How did you find out that it's not this way?

Student: From spending time in hospitals, from spending time with other doctors, from seeing many degrees of realities of it, the fact it's not free from bureaucracy and politics that are played in a lot of fields. The fact that a lot of people that are interested are in it for a lot of the wrong reasons. . . . (Field notes: Winter, third year).

The transformation from an idealistic phase to what they believe is a more realistic one occurs as students develop a professional self-image and begin to take on the identity of doctors. Accounting for this transition, one student claims:

. . . first of all, the exposure to what really goes on. You sort of keep your eyes open and you really get an idea of the real world of medicine. . . . The other part of it is when you're allowed responsibility . . . and you really become involved with patients (Field notes: Spring, second year).

Advanced students are less vocal in their questioning and criticisms of the medical profession. They attribute many of their earlier concerns to naiveté and argue for a more sympathetic view of doctors and profession:

You go through a sort of stage of disillusion in which you sort of expect doctors to be perfect, and the medical profession and treatment and everything else to be perfect. And you find out that it's not. So you sort of react to that. I think now, after about two years, I'm starting to get to the phase now where I'm quite pleased with it really. . . . Part of the flack that you hear about medical doctors and malpractice suits, and about things that go wrong, are partly due to the fact that doctors tend to look after themselves and examine their own profession very carefully (Interview: Spring, third year).

In brief, the students' shift from an idealistic perspective to one closer aligned with the realities of professional practice is accompanied by a change in the way they view and treat patients. Their priorities change as they learn how to negotiate their way through the program successfully, and they adopt the profession's rationales for treating patients as objects.

Their gradual identification and creeping commitment with the profession's ideas and ways are not, however, without serious inner struggles about the sacrifice of their idealistic views. A student pensively remarks:

> . . . they want us to be like them. I'm not sure I want to be like them. . . . We're supposed to get over our anxiety and be expressing confidence and certainty about ourselves, but how can you? On the one hand they want us to relate to patients humanly and, on the other hand, they want us to act very authoritatively. I think that's a contradiction (Field notes: Spring, second year).

This student succinctly expresses the expected alienation and separation from lay society that characterizes professionalization and lies at the heart of the objectification of clients. The process of isolation, separation, and elevation provides the context for personal change. The move towards authoritativeness in fateful matters is accompanied by external (symbolic) and internal (psychosocial) changes.

Just as the profession provides ideological justifications for changing personal values, it also helps the newcomers reshape their perceptions of what is expected and and how to "cope with" the professionalizing situation. It also provides external symbols of differentiation—thus combining a symbolic and a psychosocial separation and control. Professional symbols are crucial in reinforcing the distancing of the neophyte from lay culture and client identification.

The use and manipulation of medicine's symbol system of "medspeak" or "McBabble," the wearing of professional costume, the bearing of professional tools and props, and the management of proper performance, rituals and demeanor help differentiate and separate students from others and provide professionally appropriate ways of maintaining effective control of medical situations (Haas and Shaffir, 1982).

The symbolic cloak complements and reinforces the psychological cloak. Both, in turn, are ideologically supported and justified. Thus both ideology and symbols are critical to the waning of idealism; it is supplanted by a professionally controlled construct of reality that uses moral and actual symbols to reinforce the idea of special trustworthiness (Gerth and Mills, 1953; Kamens, 1977). A student describes the intimate connection between the professional objective of affective neutrality and the symbolic communication of competence and control when he says:

> I think that there are two things. One is that you want to establish some kind of trust between you and the patient and in order to do that you try to look cool. The other thing that comes here is that in order to actually help the patient you have to be cool. Because of those two things you try not to let your emotions interfere.

The elevation of the professional to a position of trust and control over fateful matters involves performances facilitated by a monopoly over symbols and ideas for defining the situation. The manipulation and use of these professional symbols and ideas strengthens the performance. This, in turn, convinces both outsiders and insiders, indeed the performer as well, that the professional has the situation under control. The profession-client relationship depends on trust that is ironically granted those who effectively mystify the situation and thus maintain control over uncertaintly. The symbolic/ritual process reinforces the idea of special powers, professional control over the situation, and psychological control. Thus we observe the intimate relationship between ritual drama, professional power and psychological distancing and control.

## CONCLUSION

Becoming professional involves a symbolic, ideological, and psychological transformation. In medical school, psychological separation and alienation from clients is presented to the neophyte as part of professionalization that is necessary to learning from the material (patients); to develop a trustworthy competence; to practice the profession effectively and competently by presenting an image of affective neutrality; and, to protecting the feelings of the professional by the development of a protective shield objectifiying reality.

Idealism is thus fated to change to "objective" affective neutrality as newcomers perceive and adapt to professionalizing expectations. The taking on and manipulation of professional symbols and ideas reinforces the neophytes' self-separation from lay culture and further inhibits identification with clients because of "professed" differences. The constructed inequality of the professional-client relationship undercuts newcomer idealism, and as newcomers become separated, distinguished bearers of moral authority, they must adopt both inner and outer shields. The outer shield of symbols and ideology protects them from any audience perceptions that "the emperor has no clothes." The inner carapace separates and protects the performer from emotions between equals and between conscience, feelings and "expected" behavior or proper displays of professionalism.

# Chapter VII

# *Conclusion*

As we have indicated, professionalization is best understood as a social process of legitimation of authority. This process, as has been already noted, is not just peculiar to the practice of medicine. A profession seeks to convince specific audiences or significant others that it has acquired socially desirable qualities or characteristics (Montagna, 1977; Ritzer, 1977; Wilensky, 1964). A particular occupational group makes claims to have certain socially beneficial skills and knowledge. Society accepts the claim by giving the occupational group an official mandate, or monopoly. Montagna (1977:203) aptly describes a profession's motto as "Credat Emptor"—let the buyer believe in us. Because the efficacy of a profession is difficult to evaluate, belief plays an important role in establishing a societal consensus (Etzioni, 1975; Wilensky, 1964).

The profession of medicine is a particularly useful one for analyzing the symbolic-ideological nature of the legitimating process that is so important to the professionalization of its members. To some large degree this is due to the existence of a situation that is peculiar to the practice of medicine: medicine embraces both the aspect of practical knowledge and also a belief in the profession's magical and spiritual powers. Thus, medicine is afforded a unique prestige (Larson, 1977:38–39; Siegler and Osmond, 1973) based on technical expertise enhanced by a mystique which reflects faith in power to heal. It is this dual role afforded the physician which induces the patient to grant him his trust, and hence legitimates the doctor's claim to the art and science of healing. A doctor's technical competence underpins his legitimation in a scientific sense. However, overriding this is a large component of artistry which legitimates the more subjective element essential to the diagnostic process which involves the effective use of interpersonal skills (Reuschmeyer, 1964:20).

During the course of our research, we were particularly struck by two related problems that medical students experienced in the professionalization process. Students, particularly the ones in the innovative program, experienced great uncertainty and anxiety, with the need to convince legitimating audiences by carefully manipulating symbols, ideas and people. This was a problem that had to be met and effectively managed early in the socialization process peculiar to the profession. As we sought out support for these two related ideas we came to recognize certain characteristic features of the professionalization process and thus our model emerged.

The nontraditional socialization context we studied that heightens the uncertainty of its passagees serves to give the interactional basis of reputational control and legitimation a quality which is dramatic in nature. The uncertainty, exacerbated by a nontraditional curriculum with its emphasis on interpersonal evaluation, gives primacy to the professionalizing adaptation of a cloak of competence. The form or "hidden curriculum" of professionalization is observed to be as crucial to convincing legitimating audiences as is the nature of the accompanying socialization. As students of the innovative school learn to adopt and manipulate the symbols of their profession, they create an imagery as being authoritative. During the same process, it is noted, they used to cloak and hence shut down their own feelings in respect to the more emotional demands of their chosen career.

Thus, the ritual drama of professionalization or professional socialization is organized in such a way as to convince outside legitimators and the newcomers themselves that they are being specially prepared and tested before being accorded professional status and responsibility. The process is a rigorous one—ordeal being its central and necessary feature. Newcomers are expected to experience trauma about the awesome nature of their task in preparing for future responsibility. The trials, tribulations and stresses that surround the uncertainties characteristic of status passage creates an expected and even necessary response of anxiety which the newcomer must ultimately control. Given the unique prestige that characterizes the art and practice of medicine, client expectations are often exaggerated. However, this does not mean that these expectations should not be seen to be met. Thus, the successful negotiation of the status passage must involve the projection of convincing performances that attest to the professional's competent trustworthiness. The transformation cannot be considered complete until the new professional can project an image of knowing confidence, despite any conflicting doubts about his possible inadequacies. It is through successful management of such performances that the neophyte physician is enabled to convince clients and significant others that he/she can be trusted to ease their transition towards moral, physical and/or spiritual well-being.

We began our exploration of the professionalization process by observing, and subsequently analyzing the admissions process. We noted the extreme care with which biographies were constructed and reconstructed, in order that successful applicants could idealize themselves in the face of fierce competition with many other equally worthy aspirants. Letters of admission were carefully crafted to meet gatekeeper expectations. Such letters suggested appropriate experience, ability and motivation for professionalization in the innovative program. Applicants who successfully managed this stage of the process, then prepared themselves for the interview by creating a relevant and flexible presentation of the self. Their subsequent performance in the simulated tutorial was observed as a further attempt to distinguish successful candidates by the manner in which they worked in group contexts on problem solving assignments. In sum, successful candidates demonstrate they can fit in and meet diverse and uncertain expectations from significant others.

After describing and analyzing the admissions process, we turned our attention to the uncertainties which characterize the taking on of the professional's role. We noted that some aspects of uncertainty were exacerbated by features peculiar to the innovative program. Students collectively perceived a situation fraught with high levels of stress related to meeting both immediate and long term expectations. They faced a career long process of shaping others' perceptions of their reputations. This process was central to their legitimation as a professional. Students worked hard and long to meet expectations that were not only unclear, but, in some circumstances, ambiguous.

To protect themselves from negative evaluations, rumor and gossip, neophyte students present a persona designed to please legitimating audiences. This adopted persona must also reflect a willingness to conform to the basic tenets that define the professional's role.

Then we moved to an examination of the professionalization process as it is intensified in the clinical setting. It was observed that during clerkship, the subordinate clerk, as "clinical jerk," demonstrates a heightened sensitivity to the importance of impression management. The entire process takes the form of a ritual ordeal, an initiation into a secret society where a "hidden curriculum" of adaptive behavior is developed. This is especially true of adaptive mechanisms developed as a response to feelings of uncertainty. The need to develop and project an appropriate image of trustworthiness is paramount at this stage of the professionalizing process.

At the same time that students take on an externally projected persona, a cloak of competence, which is supported by the symbols and ideas of the profession, they undergo an inner transformation whereby they learn to contain their inner feelings. It is in this way they learn to handle the difficult identification with the more sensitive areas of their experience. They learn to objectify reality, first in their need and desire to learn medicine and then, in their perceived need to demonstrate their trustworthiness to those they must emulate and who are critical to the successful advancement of their career. As they progress, they come to adopt their profession's ideology. The adaptation is that the advancing student act appropriately. Clients, it is believed, both expect and are well-served by such an approach.

We conclude by noting that neophyte idealism is fated to change because of the necessary separation and elevation of the newcomer to the role of moral authority. The external changes reflected in the successful adoption (including the manipulation of symbols and ideas) help neophytes control the definition of the situation. The internal or psychological changes help them maintain a position of affective neutrality in the face of difficult and sensitive human concerns. The successful adoption of the inner and outer cloak protects the individual from feelings and problems of transference between equals, in addition to aiding their conversion and transformation into moral authority.

We argue that idealism is fated to change as a consequence of professionalization, no matter how it is organized, because of the perceived expectations that surround the professional role. The medical profession's emphasis on an ideology of scientific and "affective neutrality" lies at the core of this structured change, but so also does the ordeal and performance character of professionalization. The pressures of time and work that the profession correlates with becoming a good and committed professional serve the "professed" ideals of service and reinforce the monopoly claims of the occupation. The good professional is the dedicated one who presumably sacrifices other interests to the exaggerated needs and demands of the special status. The emphasis on scientific and affective neutrality also strengthen the "professed" claims of special trustworthiness and competence. Thus, the monopoly interests of the profession and the context of audience legitimation of these claims require newcomers to demonstrate their commitment through the sacrifice of time and other interests. Also required is for them to move to an attitude of "detached concern" as part of their reflection of a scientific and objective perspective.

Aspirants to the professional role must communicate the service ideal as part of the "vocabulary of motives" (Mills, 1940) of the profession. This ideology of altruism, a desire to help and serve others, is altered with professionalization as the newcomer learns that caring for others is best served by detachment and objectivity. The idealism is thus reformulated from personal feelings of empathy and concern to emotional distancing and scientific rationality. The emotional involvement and identification of the neophyte with those being helped is shunted down because of the profession's belief that feelings may interfere with effective and competent service and credible performance. Professional dominance depends on control over definitions of the situation and control over definitions is served by mystification and demonstrations of the professional's self-control.

In contrasting innovative and traditional professional programs, we observe that student perceptions of what is expected of them is essentially the same. The dominance of these perceived expectations of professionalization and the uncertainty that characterized the conversion process of lay person to professional, combines to lead students in both settings to develop a common adaptation. The process by which students are resocialized and reconstituted into professional roles and statuses of power and prestige, requires they adapt their behavior in accordance with others' expectations. Among other strategies, such expectations are met by role-playing to impress evaluators.

In our focus on the professional evaluation of neophyte competence we observe that students collectively adopt strategies to meet the specific form of evaluation they encounter. In professionalizing settings that are differentially organized, we note the similarity in professional student adaptations to evaluation. When evaluation involves passing written tests, students attempt to delimit and learn the material for which they will be held accountable. When evaluation is face-to-face, students attempt to manage the impression of competence that others receive. Both written and interactional forms of evaluation of professionalizing competence involve the development by students of strategies to control the impressions significant others have of their developing competence.

Our findings corroborate other findings of the ineffectiveness of educational innovation for significant change in the process or the product of socialization. The reasons are quite similar. Educational change must alter the existing social systems, expectations and relationships. These changes must be introduced and supported in a thorough way. In the absence of consensus and shared expectations by those who control the socialization process, particularly faculty, innovation has little impact in altering the process or the product. In order for innovation to make a practical difference in the kind of graduate produced, the expectations that students perceive must be altered in a consistent way (Fullan, 1972).

The professionalization process, then, is one in which the

neophyte starts out without the means of exercising any power over his situation. As Ernest Becker (1975) argues, such a situation is adapted to by the reaching out for symbols of security and authority. The professional, in his search for security, grasps the symbolic-ideological cloak of competence to gain a measure of control—not only social control of others but also to gain control of the self. As neophytes assume the mantle of professional responsibility which commands the necessary respect, they gain a concomitant authority in fateful matters. Thus they move from an experience of total powerlessness to a position of being able to exert professional control over the lives of their clients. In the case of medicine, students move from powerlessness to Aesculapian authority (Siegler and Osmond, 1973). The process is a liminal one, characterized by dialectical extremes, and resembles the passage of an initiate into a secret society (Turner, 1970). The initiation ritual, the ordeal, the oath, the myth or legend that supports the secrecy, are all distinguishing marks of secret societies (Mackenzie, 1967:13). The route the neophyte chooses in taking on his professional role and identity is based on the learning of his occupation's secrets (Hughes, 1959), allowing him or her to conform to necessary professionalizing or reputation-making expectations. In the secret society those who share the secret share a trust, and an ensuing sense of comraderie, in the face of collective notions of professional respectability and authoritativeness.

The success, control and the subsequent gaining of a monopoly over a group's or profession's secrets and the ensuing symbolic-ideological separation and elevation to a privileged status provides the context for the paradoxical nature of the legitimating audience's reactions of trust and cynicism about "professed" competencies.

The dramatic nature of professional activity is perhaps most apparent to neophytes as they learn to manipulate the symbols and controlling ideas of their profession: they must learn to role play, and live their new identities in order to conform to the image demanded by their profession. This process has much to do with their gaining appropriate reputations of being both comptent and trustworthy. The process of conforming to, and controlling gatekeepers and others' expectations of them, typically, produces graduates who realize that success in their chosen occupation involves processes based on carefully managed interpersonal interactions with significant others.[1]

The concept of a profession as possessing the attributes of a "secret society" is neither new, nor is it meant to be understood in a pejorative sense. The analogy, based on our "findings," derives from medical students' perceptions of, and adaptations to, the ritual process of professionalization. It should also be noted that the model, emphasizing the adoption of a symbolic ideological cloak of competence, is one that characterizes professionals of other times and places. Just as there are special and secret rites that determine the structure of all secret societies, so the creation of a special class and the granting of the privileged title of physician to an individual involves a similar process. Because the clients associate the process of healing with magical power, it is not surprising that the rites de passage of the neophyte doctor into fully-fledged physician requires that he/she manipulate the symbols, ideas, ritual, myth and legends that society-at-large identify with their privileged role of healer.[2]

The most important observation in terms of the professionalization process we have explored in this study, involves, above all, the adoption of a symbolic-ideological cloak of competence, suited to convince significant audiences of the legitimacy of the professed claim of competence in serious matters. The symbolic nature of this legitimation process and the collaborative need for creating and maintaining definitions of professionalism is summarized by Gerth and Mills:

> The symbols which (thus) justify a social structure or an institutional order are called 'symbols of legitimation', or 'master symbols' or 'symbols of justification'. . . . Those in authority within institutions and social structures attempt to justify their rule by linking it, as if it were a necessary consequence, with moral symbols, sacred emblems, or legal formula which are widely believed and deeply internalized. . . . In the experience of men enacting the roles of their time, they seem (not merely correct opinions) but inevitable categories of the human mind (1953:276–277).

Professionalization as a process, then, must be understood in the context of carefully managed interactions. Clients (indeed the public at large) expect, if not demand, authoritative performances from individuals affecting the healing process. Thus it is that neophyte and practicing professionals perceive the inherent need to take on a cloak of competence in order to meet legitimating audience expectations. Professionalization thus requires symbolic-interactional and ideological control, legitimation and identification. Therein lies the crux of the process of professionalization which necessitates an alienation from the self and from others. A profession which creates exaggerated demands in a client, concomitantly, produces exaggerated work adaptations in the participant. The model we have developed in this work we feel might, profitably, be applied to all occupations that demand a trustworthy competence on the part of the client.

# Methodological Appendix

At one time field work was rooted in an oral tradition: information was passed on via a student-mentor relationship. This situation is not the case today: increasingly the methodology of field work is examined, codified and communicated in a published form.[1] This development helps meet the "need for working students in sociology to communicate the procedures and strategies of field research they have found consequential in their own studies to the less instructed or less experienced" (Habenstein, 1979:1). At the same time, field workers, researchers and teachers know there is no single best "cookbook" for conducting field research, or disentangling the practice of their method from social influence (Vidich et al., 1964: vii). We are correctly cautioned that field research experiences are highly variable and that approaches and guidelines must be adapted to the particular research problem and setting (Bogdan and Taylor, 1975). The interactional, situational, and ever-changing character of field work roles and relationships militates against the development of exact procedures. Hence the difficulty of delineating the "do's and don'ts" and "ropes" (Geer et al., 1968) of social research.

Ironically, field workers often focus on problematic relationships in the groups they study. At the same time, they ignore their own mistakes and problems. Understanding the research process, it seems, is viewed as peripheral to the research analysis. Such studied inattention to these issues (Hughes, 1951) creates a serious gap in understanding the process whereby researchers affect and are affected by research and researcher problems.

It is striking how much critical attention sociologists lavish on such measurement concerns as reliability and validity, while they often ignore theoretical and methodological conditions that affect their work (Golde, 1970; Riemer, 1977). Such studied inattention in social research is a serious defect in much sociology.[2] Researchers seldom "tell all" in reports of how data were collected, and this situation is readily accepted as the norm. By tacit agreement, for reasons going beyond professional ethics, sociologists do not press one another too hard for the details of the research process. This situation allows a state of "pluralistic ignorance" to exist concerning the hidden difficulties of conducting research.[3]

Paradoxically, in contrast to other methodologies, the very nature of field work requires investigators to talk about themselves. Indeed, some personal involvement must be conveyed in order to generate "closeness" to the situation as a warrant for the argument (Lofland, 1967). The researcher is required by the nature of field work, and by the legion canons of field work evidence, to describe personal involvement in the research. The researcher, however, typically presents an account that steers away from self-indulgent narration of personal experiences and feelings, theories about people, paranoid fantasies, embarrassments, and the like.[4] It would seem then that there are two types of accounts of field work: the one type brings out all that is devious in the self-indulgent nature of reflection, the other relies more strongly on the assumed neutrality of the unfortunately jargonistic nature of "science talk."

The theoretical perspective of symbolic interaction underlies our theoretical analysis and takes, as a given, the idea that the understanding of human conduct requires a consideration of the meanings and definitions which evoke that conduct. To understand the meaning of overt acts requires knowledge of the subjective ingredients and shared interpretations which lie at the base of the behavior. This study attempts an explanation of medical student behavior from their point of view, understanding their actions in terms of their referents.

The study of inner meanings presents a problem particular to the social sciences. Though scientific research requires objectivity, the social scientist must also be concerned with the critically important subjective bases of behavior. To attempt the understanding of behaviour in the absence of knowledge of the participants' definition is futile. Thus, overweaning objectivity in methods may reduce analysis to a state of sterility. If social science research does not take into account the subjects' point of view, the explanation and analysis must necessarily rest on intuition. Human action is inseparable from its context, and the meanings of acts cannot be divorced from actors' definitions.

Field study methods provided the modus operandi for the collection phase of this study. This approach includes a body of research strategies which allow the researcher to collect data by the most appropriate means. During this study we gathered data by the following methods: by collecting and briefing published materials, including newspaper and journal articles; by examining the official publications of the school organization; by conducting informal taped interviews, both with individuals and with groups, and by observing participants during their school and leisure activities from admission to graduation.

This study was conceived by three new Ph.D. sociologists recently employed at McMaster University, where the new and "innovative" medical school had recently opened. The three had already used field study methods (participant observation) in their dissertation research. Additionally, the combination of training and opportunity made the idea of a kind of *Boys in White* (Becker et al., 1961) study attractive. Although they approached the project with strong enthusiasm, it was plagued by difficulties and conflicts—both with school administrators and with difficulties of interaction among the researchers themselves. Retrospectively, however, these difficulties contributed to their understanding of professionalism and the inherent strains of competition for professional reputation and control.

The research strategy was an inductive one. It was ideally suited for discovering hypotheses and observing the relationships between several sets of behaviors involving different participants in varying groups and settings. The advantage of inductive research is that it enables the observer to construct and refine hypotheses as the research proceeds. Ideally, this process of reasoning results in a more complete understanding.

The inductive approach facilitates the acquisition of a more nearly complete conceptual framework and the recognition of the relationship of events, sequences of action, and contributing aspects of the situation. Contrasting with traditional, deductive social science research which seeks to isolate, contrast, and test variables, our own research strategy was intended to unveil events and circumstances that both preceeded and accompanied the process. It also determined the perception of these factors by the participants.

Upon completion of the data collection phase, all the transcribed field notes, interviews, memoranda, and briefed published materials were summarized and typed on five by eight cards. Each incident in the field notes was separated and paraphrased, unless there was a quote that was particularly illustrative and might be used in the write-up. These were quoted in full. Each incident was indentified by date and page number to facilitate ease of access. General categories were used to identify the material pertaining to the incident. Some of the general categories for reference that were used include: science–nonscience students; women students; faculty; learning appraoches; curriculum; idealism; evaluation; clerkship, and self-presentation.

As the researchers attempted to understand the best way in approaching the school about a proposed study, the initial step towards securing entrée was to utilize a faculty informant at the medical school. These discussions helped clarify the important constituencies, committees, and administrative personnel whose cooperation was important. At the same time, a proposal was written and submitted to the school, its representatives, and the proposed granting agency, Canada Council. (The proposal itself was carefully crafted to meet the anticipated concerns of the school and agency's reviewers).

The research proposal was initially rejected by the Canada Council. It was then redrafted and resubmitted utilizing the advice of a senior colleague who had had long service as a grant reviewer. From the beginning, we noted that much time and energy was involved in attempting to meet complaints concerning methodological bias or subjectivity. The agency reviewers wanted a much more specific proposal detailing exact procedures and hypotheses. School administrators shared concerns about the reliability of participant observation and expressed fears about evaluative findings. These fears could not be completely assuaged, and, during the course of the research, officials of the medical school moved from a position of reluctance to non-cooperation in relation to our proposed study. From the beginning, however, medical students were enthusiastic and cooperative. Their acceptance was crucial and aided access to many settings. Students provided rich, and sometimes intimate, stories of their experiences, travail, anguish and courage.

After one year's delay, the grant was awarded and permission granted to do the study. The actual research began with examining the process of the class of students we were to study. We immediately experienced confrontation and a strong sense of the begrudging cooperation of some school representatives. These early difficulties were exacerbated on the first day of the medical school term. An administrator's promise to grant us time to explain our research to the assembled class was not honored, and we were only cursorily introduced as members of the audience. We needed student cooperation and permission to attend tutorial meetings. This opportunity to gain the students' acceptance of our research was denied. Shortly thereafter, a school representative, (who was designated as our liaison person) recommended that we not seek access to tutorials for at least one month because of tutor and/or student reluctance.

To overcome these difficulties, we asked students at a class meeting for an opportunity to discuss our research. Their enthusiastic cooperation broke down the tutors' resistance. Although there may have been less than eager willingness on the part of some students and faculty, we were generally welcomed into tutorials and clinical settings. Some students and faculty were more cooperative and helpful than others. It was to our advantage that, by and large, students and faculty proved not to be an insurmountable problem.

Our methodological approach was to conduct a participant observation and interview study by observing and participating with students in the full range of their experiences—academic, clinical and social. We moved from a situation of disciplined naiveté to one in which we were sensitized, by the students, to their view of the professionalizing experience. We became, for many students, outsiders who were eager to learn what it meant to go through medical school. For some students we even became confidants with whom they could share the more personal parts of their experience. For a few students, our role was clearly therapeutic. This became apparent as they vented their anxieties and shared, in a safe situation, their reactions to the ordeal they were undergoing.

The field work process of this study took a number of different, but complementary, forms. We began the research by constantly being present in the library and cafeteria for the purposes of meeting the students. We met the class at a class meeting. There we explained our research proposal and accepted their invitation to observe Phase I tutorial groups. With the exception of the first month, our observations of tutorial and clinical experiences were non-problematic. To ensure that we did not miss any critical data, we gained access to the first month's tutorials of the following year's class. Upon completion of each observation, we dictated, in as complete and verbatim form as possible, our findings. Later these were typed and copies made.

During the research phase, informal individual and group interviews were conducted and the data recorded. During the third year of the study, we conducted intensive individual and group interviews with the students. These became increasingly structured as we began testing and receiving feedback on hypotheses and concepts that had evolved in the field.

At the end of the second year, we wrote papers on medical student anxiety and the "cloak of competence" (Haas and Shaffir, 1977). These papers were randomly distributed to students for written and oral comments. Their comments added to, and refined our ideas, and fed into the developing model of our analysis. We also sent copies of our papers to selected faculty and administrators for comments.

## THE BARGAIN RELATIONSHIP

Field researchers use such phrases as "making the bargain," "developing rapport," and "working as a team." These phrases abstract aspects of the research process. The implicit assumption is that once the bargain is made, rapport should develop. Once the team is organized, no further negotiation is necessary. Our experience tells us that these are not fixed "stages," but rather a series of continuous processes. This new conceptualization of the research served to shift our attention to the important problems of maintaining (negotiating and re-negotiating), not only establishing, research and researcher relationships.

The nature of any bargain relationship is likely to shift and alter (Johnson, 1975). What is referred to as the "bargain stage" of the research is more accurately conceptualized as a series of negotiations throughout the research endeavor wherein the researcher continually attempts to secure others' cooperation. Bargain negotiations typically require the development of relationships of equality, involving the idea of exchange, or "give and take." This is particularly true in relationships between professionals. These relationships are symbolically communicated in interaction and negotiations that indicate the development and maintenance of a collegial relationship (Strauss et al., 1964; Haas, 1972).

Our analysis focuses on negotiations with gatekeepers and also negotiations amongst ourselves. We observed that in both sets of relationships, participants' concerns with the development and maintaining professional reputations conflicted with the development and maintenance of professional collegiality. Gatekeepers of a new, innovative and internationally recognized school and young Ph.D.'s in sociology were revealed to share similar concerns about professional reputation. This situation created strains and conflicts which led to the breakdown of collegiality and cooperation.

The negotiation and renegotiations with gatekeepers and among the researchers reveal a cyclical pattern of "career." Bargains, in both relationships, were made between the participants' assuming a context of collegiality. Conflicting interests and commitments in establishing and maintaining professional reputations created strains. These difficulties were exacerbated by the development of a context of pretense awareness (Glaser and Strauss, 1964) in which parties refrained from confronting each other because of the assumption of collegiality. This context was disrupted when one party formally expressed their interests and grievances, thus challenging the veneer of collegiality and forcing a renegotiation and reconstitution of the relationship. Conflicting professional interests and commitments created difficulties for maintaining professional collegiality and agreement.

### Gatekeeper Bargains

An irreducible conflict exists between the interests of the researcher and the representatives of the organization (Becker, 1964:272–276). It is not surprising then, that organizations attempt to define, limit and control others' investigations of their activities. They want to ensure that the research is compatible with their interests and casts their activities in a favorable light. This underlying concern is likely to be aggravated when researchers examine the understructure of an institution. This is particularly apparent when that institution is highly organized and powerful (Habenstein, 1970:99–121).

We met our first problem in trying to secure a bargain with representatives of a high image profession in the context of the new and reputation-conscious school. Sociologists routinely make bargains to study people with less power, status and prestige. However, the study of the most powerful professions makes bargains based upon shared interests and collegiality inherently problematic and difficult. The professions are by definition, groups which attempt to control definitions of a situation. This control is threatened by outsiders, (such as ourselves) who observe the professionalization process first-hand. The basis of professional power and control, centers upon a process by which professionals mystify their competence. Thus, they obscure the basis of authority by providing a justification for inequality of status, closure of access, monopolization of knowledge, and control over perceptions of reality which define the situation (Haas and Shaffir, 1978; Larson, 1977). Our interests in observing the professionalization process first-hand was met by a wary, uncertain, and reluctant set of gatekeepers.

In order to receive official permission to study the socialization of medical students, we attended a series of meetings with medical school faculty, administrators and students. We prepared and submitted a proposal to examine the socialization process from the students' point-of-view. We described the theoretical underpinnings of our research and our methodology. Our discussions of the proposal in committee and in public meetings were characterized by two central gatekeeper concerns and reservations: how can a methodology lacking in "rigorous design" result in a scientifically accurate analysis; and, to what extent would our analysis make statements about program success and failure? Although we expected that our proposal would be carefully and critically examined, we did not fully anticipate the strength of the institution's reluctance to it.

From the beginning, we felt we were parties to a bargain made only reluctantly. Our first days in the field (Geer, 1964) indicated that we would continue to have problems with the gatekeepers. An agreement that we would have an opportunity to introduce ourselves, and our research, to incoming students at their first meeting was violated, hampering our early efforts and thus indicated that the relationship might not proceed smoothly.

While initial discussions with the school's administration suggested that frequent meetings would be mutually desirable, the two groups did not meet to discuss our work or any problems related to it. The relationship became characterized by "pretense awareness': that is to say both parties were aware of strains in the relationship but pretended otherwise (Glaser and Strauss, 1964). At the beginning of the third and final year of the research, we met with the school liaison person to request institutional data about the cohort we studied. Our difficult relationship was due in part to a research bargain which did not clearly identify the rights and obligations we expected. In spite of this, we presumed that such materials as admission letters and background information, (if properly treated through norms of confidentiality and anonymity) would be forthcoming. After six months without a response, we realized trouble loomed. The procrastination of the committee provided a dire warning. Yet, even our trepidation did not match the fierceness of their eventual reaction. We learned that our request had "prompted a thorough review of the entire project by members of the medical faculty."

As negotiations continued, it became apparent that the committee's fundamental concern related to our preliminary findings about the students' socialization. We believed that the committee members' comments and questions about our methodological design and the representativeness of our data were indicative of their main concerns about how our findings, analysis and model would affect the school's reputation. Faced with researchers employing, by their definition, a highly subjective methodology, and developing an analysis attaching credibility to the students' views, the committee was anxious to organize a regular exchange of views concerning both the direction and analysis of the project.

The executive committee claimed that our methodological approach lacked sufficient rigor and clarity. Consequently, they invited a methodologist affiliated with the medical school to appraise and evaluate our research design. Much to our surprise, in the midst of a meeting during which we were invited to justify our methodological orientation, an executive committee member announced that steps would immediately be taken to provide us access to the requested data. The verbal agreement stipulated that we would provide the committee with a draft of analyses containing those data.

Our relationship with the medical school gatekeepers was influenced by conflicting and changing definitions of the situation. This affected the ease with which specific data could be collected. The evolving nature of this relationship was paralleled by a changing relationship among members of the research team. Conflicting personal and professional interests and commitments, in addition to the problem of maintaining a relationship based upon collegiality, led to a process of renegotiation. This eventually caused a break-up of the research team.

### Competing Commitments and Researcher Bargains

As Douglas (1976:221) has suggested, field research traditionally involves a "Lone Ranger" approach in which the researcher works independently. Academics are socialized and rewarded primarily for individual research. Thus, they are ill-prepared for the problems and conflicts inherent in an enterprise involving joint scholarship. Team field research offers an alternative. Several researchers have spelled out the advantages offered by this kind of research. They have included among its benefits the possibilities for fuller coverage, validity, checking of generalizations, and the gaining of a multiperspectival view of society (Douglas, 1976; Pelto, 1970). Along with these advantages, the drawbacks to team field research have also been recognized (Yancey and Rainwater, 1970). Valentine argues that, "the psychological problems of field relationships between researcher and subjects are quite sufficient so that further complications in the form of interpersonal difficulties among team members should certainly be avoided (1968:181)."

A joint endeavor involving team research is a tension frought exercise in the best of circumstances. Problems arise concerning differences in theoretical and methodological perspectives, and in developing working relationships where personality conflicts are kept to a minimum. The problem of time spent on the research project became a major problem among several important conflicts (Zimmerman and Wieder, 1977). This was a problem brought to the surface during the course of our research. The pressures of our personal and professional lives minimized the possibility of scheduling regular team meetings, in which concerns and problems could be voiced and resolved. In fact, shortage of time became an important area of contention in terms of team commitment and contribution.

In our case, conflict in our three-member team resulted primarily from the additional side-bets (Becker, 1960) we were making to extablish and protect our professional careers and reputations. One of our members became involved in another research project going on at the same medical school. The researcher did not realize the extent of the necessary involvement in this project. Unfortunately, he failed to discuss the situation with the other two members of our research group. The problem was further exacerbated. At the same time, the two remaining team members agreed to edit a book. In addition, all of the research group were writing up other research for publication. In short, professional, career and family pressures led each of us to pursue alternative commitments that detracted from our joint project. Due to the longitudinal nature of our medical socialization project, we anticipated that a period of time would elapse before publication. This fact, and the pressure to publish, undermined our commitment to the project.

As a result of these conflicting priorities, we were less able than we wished to read and comment on field notes, generate memoranda, and meet together about the problems and directions of the research in question. We had difficulty finding time to read bibliographic materials which would provide support for some of the notions we were developing in the field. Meetings for maintaining collegiality, sharing and analyzing our observations, and generating new theoretical directions occurred only sporadically. In sum, conflicting interests and commitments set up barriers to communication thus compromising not only the research but the researchers themselves.

Subsequentially, in-fighting and disagreements in our own group and with the gatekeepers increased. We initially tended to down play or ignore them. Although each individual in the project was aware that we had a problem that should be addressed, indeed each member of the group was sensitive to the others' awareness, the deteriorating group dynamic was not acknowledged. In an attempt to preserve collegiality we felt impotent to assign blame, and hoped that the problem would resolve itself.

Individual and collective anxieties were only intermittently expressed. The uneven nature of our observations resulted in our developing strategies designed to assuage the self and/or others about the relative amounts of time spent in the field. We justified periods of absence from the field in the hope of gaining sympathetic understanding. Such "understanding" was almost always offered. When a group member was confronted with a similar situation, it was always reciprocated. When unable to enter the field for a period of time, we would reassure one another that the "lost time" would be recovered, even to the point of specifying precisely how this would be accomplished. Usually, however, such absences were not discussed. Each of us feared that raising the topic might lead to recriminations. The reciprocity of avoidance behavior sustained the bargain, but built up emotional strain that prevented us from facing up to the rapidly deteriorating situation. Other problems arose: differences of opinion about research roles, methods of collecting and analyzing data, and the publication and authorship of findings created further strains among the researchers. One member resorted to the writing of memorandum, in which he tabulated the number of transcribed pages of field notes dictated by each of the researchers. He was seriously questioning his further participation in the project. In frustration over his colleagues' absence from the field he wrote:

> This memo is of critical importance to my own continuing involvement in this project. . . . This situation (his coinvestigators' absence from the field) is unacceptable to me. First, I feel the situation is not just. I do not wish to carry what is ostensibly a joint project largely on my own shoulders. Secondly, I'm rapidly losing any confidence which I initially had, that the project would be successful. I am putting as much time into the project as I can and this time is not being matched by my co-participants. . . . This may sound nasty, but under these circumstances, I feel I must ask for an agreement in writing between us concerning ownership, including order of authorship of any material which is written from this project.

Use of a memo and the disruption of our "gentlemen's agreement" was resented by the others. However an ensuing discussion provided an explicit recognition of the "competing commitments" (Becker, 1960) and bargaining problem. The groundwork was laid down for a consideration of a renegotiation. We repaired relations and moved again to a "real" collegiality by developing supplementary methodological approaches to help us meet students. This allowed us to increase the amount of data gathered on a designated schedule. We thus renewed and re-expressed full commitment to the project and forestalled a more serious situation.

For a time, the pressure that led to conflict drew us together, re-emphasizing our sense of interdependence. As time passed, the side-bets we made on successful continuance of the study had accumulated. These bear enumeration. The research bargain with the medical students committed us morally to carrying out the project. Our reputations with professional colleagues, the funding agency, and the discipline's reputation within the university community were at stake. Public presentations extended our side-bets and renewed our commitment. At the same time, however, we began to hedge our bets. Rather than fully commit ourselves to a troubled project, each of us further developed alternative interests in research and teaching, thus exacerbating our competing commitments, the chief source of difficulties.

As Simmel (1950) has described them, triadic relationships are inherently stressful because of the emergence of coalitions. As the project developed, one of the researchers became isolated. He had little opportunity for interaction with the others, who had continued to meet regularly to discuss their joint work. At the start of the second year, the isolated researcher formulated a proposal to reduce his field work role. This balanced his contribution with those of his co-researchers. This proposed reduction of his input eventually led to his total withdrawal from the field to observe the seriousness of his colleagues' field work contribution. His withdrawal was another signal that irresolvable difficulties were affecting the team. The situation worsened until, in an explosive confrontation, the team was reconstituted from three to two members.

The consequences of our problems in terms of the emerging sociological model and analysis are impossible to measure. The research triad undoubtedly contributed to the mix of ideas. However, in the face of continuing conflict, the progress of this research was deterred. The breakdown of communication and collegial relations obviated the implicit value of additional theoretical input.

Once reconstituted into a group that was communicating, the research team worked successfully. The remaining members faced the pressing problem of successfully carrying out the research. This was possible only by making a new commitment to the project. United as the survivors of an unpleasant experience, the remaining researchers moved in unison to accomplish the research.

With a renewed investment in the troubled project, and the difficulties of team relations effectively resolved, the remaining members worked to observe students in their activities and were able to develop and test a model that was now emerging. Continuing collaboration with regular, usually daily, meetings about field and interview experiences, resulted in the development of an increasing confidence and excitement about the research.

## CONCLUSION

Field researchers use phrases to describe their relationships with gatekeepers, subjects, and each other. These phrases capsulize processes which culminate in desired conditions of collegiality. "Making a bargain," "developing rapport," and "working as a team" all imply phases of the research process.

The conception of the research process as having a determinate career with specific "stages" contributes to our neglect of the changing relationships that characterize all social interaction. Our research experiences allowed us to call attention to the methodological neglect of problems concerning the maintainance of field relationships. These experiences suggested that in avoiding our "mistakes at work" we limit an understanding of the research process. Researchers are obliged to describe their theories and methods, but typically do not discuss problems and mistakes. An aspect of our work is the tacit agreement to avoid focusing on the more personal aspects of our research activity. Thus we limit ourselves to concerns about how we affect research subjects (Rosenthal and Rosnow, 1970), failing to describe how we are affected by other interests, commitments, and relationships.

We have focused on two sets of professional relationships in our research that had problematic results. Concerns about professional reputation and the absence of opportunities for maintaining collegial relationships and shared definitions of the situation resulted in conflict. Because these relationships are based on the concept of collegiality, we noted the development of a context of pretense awareness. Participants perceived a changing and deteriorating relationship, but acted as if past understandings would serve as a basis for mutual cooperation. This context was disrupted in both sets of relationships by the raising of background issues by one party to the relationship. The formalization of issues produced a new situation requiring remedial attention and, ultimately, renegotiation. Competing interests and definitions of the situation created strains and conflicts that disrupted the concept of collegiality altering the basis of the relationship, and leading to a renegotiation and reconsitution of the relationship.[5]

# Notes

## Chapter I

1. The school we studied—McMaster Medical School—is located in Hamilton, Ontario, Canada. As a convenient shorthand we refer to traditional approaches to medical education in contrast to the so-called innovative approach observed in the school we studied. We realize that these approaches are ideal types. Each school shares some elements of the other (Popper, 1967) but the typical model we have in mind refers to the studies by Becker et al., 1961; Merton et al., 1957; Bloom, 1973.

2. The analyses in the introduction and conclusion of occupational professionalization are informed by the excellent seminar paper of Ms. Gail Coulas.

## Chapter III

1. For those clearly identifiable in the academic stream, the letters are of little importance. This point was clearly made by two letters from academic-stream candidates. One letter barely exceeded one double-spaced page and both were characterized by poor grammar and spelling. It was clear the letters were perfunctory exercises.

## Chapter V

1. Ernest Becker (1975) argues that man's innate and all-encompassing fear of death drives him to attempt to transcend death through culturally standardized hero systems and symbols.

2. The complaint that physicians avoid patient death and dying is partly explained in the basic human fear of death (Becker, 1975). Although they may grow more desensitized to others' death and dying, they are, at the same time, more often reminded of their own mortality. Moreover, the doctor facing such a situation of telling patient and/or family of impending death is

vulnerable to charges of incompetence or failure and it is competence or its appearance that defines the doctor's role.

3.  This reaction was not unexpected. As Merton et al. suggest in a study of a more traditional program:

> The immediate future of a medical student is largely contingent upon the appraisals of his performance by the faculty. . . . They are motivated to *know* what is expected of them by the faculty and to *know* in what measure they are meeting these expectations. . . . When the pattern of periodically reporting their grades to students is curtailed or eliminated, there apparently develops a marked concern to find substitute bases for answering the institutionally-generated question: 'how am I making out?' (1957:67–68).

4.  The process is analogous to those described among workers balancing superiors' and fellow workers' expectations. See, for example, Roethlisberger and Dickson (1939) and Roy (1952).

5.  One merely has to note the numerous and apparently increasing number of imposters who have been discovered in medical practice. See, for example, *New York Times*, February 20, 1983, p.24. See also Frank Abnagale, Jr. (1982) for a discussion of how the author posed successfully as a member of various professions.

6.  The genre of this script is certainly not unique to the professionalization of medical practitioners. For an analogous example of an occupational group that uses collective adoption of a cloak of competence to deal with anxiety about fateful matters, see Haas, 1977. See also Edgerton's analysis of mental retardates' attempts to pass in conventional society by adoption of such a cloak of competence (1967). These examples suggest that the demand for credible performance is accented in those social roles that are perceived as bearing exaggerated expectations about competence.

7.  For an example of an occupation where members shroud themselves in a cloak of competence, see Haas (1972, 1974, 1977). High steel ironworkers, like physicians, must act competently and confidently in fateful matters. Ironworker apprentices, like student-physicians, were observed attempting to control others' definitions of them by acting competently and not revealing their fear or ignorance. In both situations we find neophytes reluctant to reveal their incompetence.

8.  Ernest Becker reminds social scientists about their most important question and responsibility when he says: "How do we get rid of the power to mystify? The talent and processes of mesmerization and mystification have to be exposed. Which is another way of saying that we have to work against both structural and psychological unfreedom in society. The task of science would be to explore both of these dimensions" (1975:165). Our analysis suggests that demystification requires an appreciation of the interactive, collaborative and symbolic nature of professional-client relations and definitions of the situation.

## Chapter VI

1.   Although this chapter focuses on the reformulation and/or loss of the students' idealistic perspective, it is important to realize that students' decisions to enter medicine reflect different and competing perspectives. The idealistic perspective is, however, the one most frequently and consistently articulated by the students we followed. One can suggest the interesting possibility that idealism may be understood as a convenient "vocabulary of motives" (Mills, 1940) accounting for career choice and may be seen as part of the profession's ideology emphasizing the "service ideal." By implication, idealism is then actually created by the desire to study medicine and its subsequent loss or transformation is part of medical ideology. We argue that loss of idealism is inherent in professionalization, but this is not to deny that students may enter medicine with a sense of idealism desiring to approach and treat people humanistically.

## Chapter VII

1.   See Victor Turner (1970) for a description of the time-honored process of liminality. The moral transformation experienced by professionalizing students, involving mortification and degradation, is similar to the moral transformation of stigma encountered by the person labeled as deviant (Garfinkel, 1956; Goffman, 1963). Both neophyte professionals and deviants are involved in a moral transformation whereby they are converted into a new master status and identity.

2.   As professed bearers of special knowledge and expertise, professionals lay claim to special responsibilities and autonomy which, in the case of medicine, Freidson (1970) and others (Mendelson, 1979; Siegler and Osmond (1973) have analyzed as a state religion having an "officially approved monopoly of the right to define health and illness and to treat illness" (Freidson, 1970:5).

## METHODOLOGICAL APPENDIX

1.   For example, see: Becker, 1970; Bogdan and Taylor, 1975; Douglas, 1976; Filstead, 1970; Golde, 1970; Habenstein, 1970; Hammond, 1964; Johnson, 1975; Junker, 1960; Lofland, 1971, 1976; Powdermaker, 1966; Schatzman and Strauss, 1973; Shaffir, et al., 1980; Shipman, 1976; and Vidich et al., 1964.

2.   For the most part, there has been little public discussion of the subjective aspects of field work. Although sociology contains an enormous literature on the subject, Robert K. Merton noted some time ago that it is primarily concerned with how social scientists ought to think, feel and act and fails to draw necessary attention to what they actually do, think, and feel (1962:19). There are, however, exceptions and a number of researchers have provided

personal chronicles of their research in which they have focused attention on the process of interaction between the researcher and community members, and on the personal considerations affecting both the organization and outcome of their research activity. Some of the better ones include: Gans, 1968; Golde, 1970; Habenstein, 1970; Hammond, 1964; Johnson, 1975; Leibow, 1967; Roth, 1966; Vidich, Bensman and Stein, 1964; Watson, 1969; and Whyte, 1955.

3.    Professionals typically overlook questions of peer competency and evaluation focuses around matters of presentation and tact. Professional competency tends to take the form of a "gentleman's agreement" which sustains the "taken-for-granted" definition of the situation. This reality is sustained by symbolic demonstrations of competence. On this general point see Freidson, 1975, Ch.8; Haas and Shaffir, 1977; Light, 1972; Millman, 1976; and the classic statement by E.C. Hughes on "mistakes at work" (1951b). On the concept of pluralistic ignorance, see Schanck, 1932:102, 130–131; Mayer and Rosenblatt, 1975.

4.    We are indebted to Prue Rains for making this point.

5.    The stages involved in negotiation and renegotiation of our research and researcher relationships generally parallel the insightful conceptualization of negotiations of teacher-pupil and teacher-teacher interactions by Martin, 1976.

# References

Abnagale, F., Jr.
    1982    *Catch Me If You Can.* New York: Pocket Books.
Apple, M.
    1971    "The hidden curriculum and the nature of conflict." *Interchange* 2:27–40.
Ball, D.
    1967    "The ethnography of an abortion clinic." *Social Problems* 14:293–301.
Becker, Ernest
    1975    *Escape from Evil.* New York: The Free Press.
Becker, H.S.
    1960    "Notes on the concept of commitment." *American Journal of Sociology* 66:32–40
    1962    "The nature of a profession." Pp.27–46 in *Education for the Professions,* Sixty-first Yearbook of the National Society for the Study in Education, Part II. University of Chicago Press.
    1964    "Problems in the publication of field studies." Pp.267–284 in Vidich, Arthur J., Joseph Bensman, and Maurice R. Stein (eds.) *Reflections on Community Studies.* New York: John Wiley and Sons.
Becker, H.S. and B. Geer
    1958    "The fate of idealism in medical school." *American Sociological Review* 23: 50–56.
Becker, H.S., B. Geer, E.C. Hughes, and A.L. Strauss
    1961    *Boys in White: Student Culture in Medical School.* Chicago: University of Chicago Press.
Becker, H.S., B. Geer and E.C. Hughes
    1968    *Making the Grade: The Academic Side of College Life.* New York: John Wiley and Sons.
Blankenship, R.L. (ed.)
    1977    *Colleagues in Organizations: The Social Construction of Professional Work.* New York: John Wiley and Sons.

Bloom, S.
1973     *Power and Dissent in the Medical School.* New York: Macmillan.

Bogdan R. and S.J. Taylor
1975     *Introduction to Qualitative Research Methods: A Phenomenological Approach to the Social Sciences.* New York: John Wiley.

Bourdieu, P.
1973     "Cultural reproduction and social reproduction." Pp.71–112. R. Brown (ed.) *Knowledge, Education, and Cultural Change.* London: Tavistock.

Bramson, R.
1973     "The secularization of American medicine." *Hastings Center Studies* 1: 17–28.

Broadhead, R.
1983     *The Private Lives and Professional Identity of Medical Students.* New Brunswick, N.J.: Transaction, Inc.

Bucher, R. and J. Stelling
1977     *Becoming Professional.* Beverly Hills, CA: Sage.

Collins, R.
1982     *Sociological Insight: An Introduction to Non-Obvious Sociology.* New York: Oxford University Press.

Coombs, R.H.
1978     *Mastering Medicine: Professional Socialization in Medical School.* New York: Macmillan.

Coombs, R.H. and B.P. Boyle
1971     "The transition to medical school: expectations versus realities." Pp.91–109 in R.H. Coombs and C.E. Vincent (eds.) *Psychosocial Aspects of Medical Training.* Springfield, Ill.: Charles C. Thomas.

Coombs, R.H. and P.S. Powers
1975     "Socialization for death: the physician's role." *Urban Life* 4: 250–271.

Davis, F.
1968     "Professional socialization as subjective experience: the process of doctrinal conversion among student nurses." Pp.235–251 in H.S. Becker et al. (eds.) *Institutions And The Person.* Chicago: Aldine Publishing Company.

Daniels, M.J.
1960     "Affect and its control in the medical intern." *American Journal of Sociology* 66: 259–267.

Douglas, J.
1976     *Investigative Social Research: Individual and Team Field Research.* Beverly Hills, CA: Sage.

Edgerton, R.B.
1967     *The Cloak of Competence: Stigma In The Lives Of The Mentally Retarded.* Berkeley: University of California Press.

Emerson, J.P.
1970     "Behavior in private places: sustaining definitions of reality in

gynecological examinations." Pp.73–97 in H.P. Dreitzel (ed.) *Recent Sociology*. New York: The Macmillan Company.

Etzioni, A.
1975    *A Comparative Analysis of Complex Organizations: On Power, Involvement and their Correlates*. New York: The Free Press.

Filstead, W. (ed.)
1970    *Qualitative Methodology: Firsthand Involvement with the Social World*. Chicago: Markham.

Fox, R.
1957    "Training for uncertainty." Pp.207–241 in Robert K. Merton, George G. Reader and Patricia L. Kendal (eds.) *The Student Physician*. Cambridge, Mass.: Harvard University Press.

1974    "Is there a 'new' medical student?" Pp.197–227 in L.R. Tancred (ed.) *Ethics of Health Care*. Institute of Medicine: National Academy of Science.

Fredericks, M.A. and P. Mundy
1976    *The Making of a Physician*. Chicago: Loyola University Press.

Freidson, E.
1970    *Profession of Medicine*. New York: Dodds Mead and Company.
1975    *Doctoring Together*. New York: Elsevier.

Fullan, M.
1972    "Overview of the innovative process and the user." *Interchange* 3:1–46.

Gans, H.
1968    "The participant-observer as a human being: observations on the personal aspects of field work." Pp.300–317 in H.S. Becker et al (eds.) *Intitutions And The Person*. Chicago: Aldine.

Garfinkel, H.
1956    "Conditions of successful degradation ceremonies: *American Journal of Sociology* 61:420–424.

Geer, B.
1964    "First days in the field." Pp.322–344 in Hammond, P. (ed.) *Sociologists at Work: Essays on the Craft of Social Research*. Garden City, N.Y.: Doubleday Company.

1972    *Learning to Work*. Beverly Hills, CA: Sage Publications, Inc.

Geer, B., J. Haas, C. Vivona, S.J. Miller, C. Woods, and H.S. Becker
1968    "Learning the ropes: situational learning in four occupational training programs." Pp.209–233 in I. Deutscher and E.J. Thompson (eds.) *Among the People: Encounters with the Poor*. New York: Basic Books, Inc.

Gerth, H. and C.W. Mills
1953    *Character and Social Structure: The Psychology of Social Institutions*. New York: Harcourt, Brace, Jovanovich.

Glaser, B. and A.L. Strauss
1964    "Awareness contexts and social interaction." *American Sociological Review* 29:669–679.

1971    *Status Passage*. Chicago: Aldine.

Goffman, E.
1959    *The Presentation of Self in Everyday Life*. Garden City, N.Y.: Double-
        day-Anchor.
1961    *Asylums*. New York: Doubleday
1963    *Stigma: Notes on the Management of Spoiled Identity*. Baltimore:
        Penguin.
Golde, P. (ed.)
1970    *Women in the Field: Anthropological Experiences*. Chicago: Aldine.
Goode, W.J.
1957    "Community within a community: the professions." *American Soci-
        ological Review* 22:194–200.
Haas, J.
1972    "Binging: educational control among high-steel ironworkers."
        *American Behavioral Scientist* 16:27–34.
1974    "The stages of the high-steel ironworker apprentice career." *The
        Sociological Quarterly* 15:93–108.
1977    "Learning real feelings: a study of high-steel ironworkers' reac-
        tions to fear and danger." *Sociology of Work and Occupations* 4:147–
        170.
Haas, J. and W. Shaffir
1978    "Do new ways of professional socialization make a difference?: a
        study of professional socialization." Paper presented at the Ninth
        World Congress of Sociology, Uppsala, Sweden.
1977    "The professionalization of medical students: developing compe-
        tence and a cloak of competence." *Symbolic Interaction* 1:71–88.
1982a   "Taking on the role of doctor: a dramaturgical analysis of pro-
        fessionalization." *Symbolic Interaction* 5:187–203.
1982b   "Ritual evaluation of competence: the hidden curriculum of
        professionalization in an innovative medical school program."
        *Work and Occupations* 9:131–154.
Haas, J., V. Marshall and W. Shaffir
1981    "Initiation into medicine: neophyte uncertainty and the ritual
        ordeal of professionalization." Pp. 109–123 in L. Lundy and B.
        Warme (eds.) *Work in the Canadian Context: Continuity Despite
        Change*. Toronto: Butterworths.
Habenstein, R.
1970    *Pathways to Data: Field Methods for Studying Ongoing Social Organiza-
        tions*. Chicago: Aldine.
Halmos, P.
1970    *The Personal Service Society*. New York: Schocken.
Henslin, J.
1968    "Trust and the cab driver." Pp. 138–158 in M. Truzzi (ed.) *Soci-
        ology and Everyday Life*. Englewood Cliffs, N.J.: Prentice-Hall.
Hamilton, J.D.
1972    "The selection of medical students at McMaster University." *Jour-
        nal of the Royal College of Physicians of London* 6: 348–351.

Hammond, P. (ed.)
    1964    *Sociologists at Work: Essays on the Craft of Social Research.* Garden
            City, N.Y.: Doubleday and Company.
Hughes, E.C.
    1945    Dilemmas and contradictions of status." *American Journal of Soci-*
            *ology* 50:353–359.
    1951a   "Work and self." Pp. in J.H. Rohrer and M. Sherif (eds.) *Social*
            *Psychology at the Crossroads.* New York: Harper & Row.
    1951b   "Mistakes at work." *Canadian Journal of Economics and Political*
            *Science* 17: 320–327.
    1952    "The sociological study of work: an editorial foreward." *The Amer-*
            *ican Journal of Sociology* 62.
    1956    "The making of a physician." *Human Organization* 14: 21–25.
    1959    "The study of occupations." Pp. in R.K. Merton, L. Broom, and
            L.S. Cottrell, Jr. (eds.) *Sociology Today.* New York: Basic Books.
    1963    "Professions." *Daedalus* 92 (Fall): 655–658.
Johnson, J.
    1975    *Doing Field Research.* New York: Free Press.
Junker, B.
    1960    *Field Work: An Introduction to the Social Sciences.* Chicago: Univer-
            sity of Chicago Press.
Kadushin, C.
    1962    "Social distance between client and professional." *American Jour-*
            *nal of Sociology* 67:517–531.
Kamens, D.H.
    1977    "Legitimating myths and educational organization: the rela-
            tionship between organizational ideology and formal structure."
            *American Sociological Review* 42:208–219.
Larson, M.S.
    1977    *The Rise of Professionalism: A Sociological Analysis.* Berkeley: Univer-
            sity of California Press.
Leeson, J. and J. Gray
    1978    *Women and Medicine.* London: Tavistock Publications.
Liebow, E.
    1976    *Tally's Corner.* Boston: Little, Brown and Company.
Lief, H.I. and R. Fox
    1963    "Training for 'detached concern' in medical students." Pp. 12–35
            in H.I. Lief et al. (eds.) *The Psychological Basis of Medical Practice.*
            New York: Harper & Row.
Light, D.W. Jr.
    1972    "Psychiatry and suicide: the management of a mistake." *American*
            *Journal of Sociology* 77: 821–383.
    1980    *Becoming Psychiatrists: The Professional Transformation of Self.* New
            York: W.W. Norton and Company.
Lofland, J.
    1967    "Notes on naturalism in sociology." *Kansas Journal of Sociology*
            3:45–61.

1971    *Analyzing Social Settings: A Guide to Qualitative Observation and Analysis.* Belmont, CA: Wadsworth.

1976    *Doing Social Life: The Qualitative Study of Human Interaction in Natural Settings.* New York: Wiley.

Lortie, D.
1968    "Shared ordeal and induction to work." Pp.252–264 in H.S. Becker et al. (eds.) *Institutions And The Person.* Chicago: Aldine.

Mackenzie, N.
1962    *Secret Societies.* New York: Holt, Rinehart and Winston.

Mayer, J.E. and A. Rosenblatt
1975    "Encounters with danger: social workers in the ghetto." *Sociology of Work and Occupations* 2: 227–245.

Martin, W.B.
1976    *The Negotiated Order of the School.* Toronto: Macmillan of Canada.

Maurer, D.
1962    *The Big Con.* New York: New American Library.

Mechanic, D.
1962    *Students Under Stress: A Study in the Social Psychology of Adaptation.* New York: Macmillan.

Mendelsohn, R.
1979    *Confessions of a Medical Heretic.* Chicago: Contemporary Books.

Merton, R.K., G.C. Reader and P.L. Kendall (eds.)
1957    *The Student Physician.* Cambridge, MA: Harvard University Press.

Millman, M.
1976    *The Unkindest Cut.* New York: William Morrow.

Mills, C.W.
1940    Situated actions and vocabularies of motive." *American Sociological Review* 5:904–913.

Montagna, P.D.
1977    "The professions: approaches to their study." Pp. 195–219 in P.D. Montagna *Occupations and Society: Toward a Sociology of the Labor Market.* New York: John Wiley.

Neufeld, V.R. and H.S. Barrows
1974    "The 'McMaster philosophy': an approach to medical education." *Journal of Medical Education* 49: 1040–1050.

Oakley, A.
1976    "Wisewoman and medicine man: changes in the management of childbirth." Pp.17–58 in J. Mitchell and A. Oakley (eds.) *The Rights and Wrongs of Women.* Middlesex: Penguin Books.

Olesen, V.L. and E.W. Whittaker
1968    *The Silent Dialogue: A Study in the Social Psychology of Professional Socialization.* San Francisco: Jossey-Bass.

Orth, C.D. III
1963    *Social Structure and Learning Climate: The First Year at the Harvard Business School.* Boston: Division of Research, Graduate School of Business Administration, Harvard University.

Parsons, T.
1951    *The Social System.* London: Routledge & Kegan Paul.

Pelto, P.J.
1970    *Anthropological Research.* New York: Harper & Row.

Popper, H. (ed.)
1967    *Trends in Medical Schools.* New York: Grune and Stratton.

Postman, N. and C. Weingartner
1969    *Teaching as a Subversive Activity.* New York: Dell Publishing Co.

Powdermaker, H.
1966    *Stranger and Friend: The Way of an Anthropologist.* New York: W.W. Norton & Company, Inc.

Prus, R. and C.D. Sharper
1979    *Road Hustler.* Toronto: Gage.

Riemer, J.W.
1977    "Varieties of opportunistic research." *Urban Life and Culture* 5:461–477.

Ritzer, G.
1977    *Working: Conflict and Change.* Second Edition. Englewood Cliffs, N.J.· Prentice-Hall, Inc.

Roethlisberger, F.J. and W.J. Dickson
1939    *Management and the Worker.* Cambridge, MA: Harvard University Press.

Ross, A.D.
1961    *Becoming a Nurse.* Toronto: Macmillan Company of Canada.

Roth, J.
1957    "Ritual and magic in the control of contagion." *American Sociological Review* 22:310–314.

1966    "Hired hand research." *American Sociologist* 1: 190–196.

Roy, D.
1952    "Quota restriction and goldbricking in a machine shop." *American Journal of Sociology* 57:427–a442.

Rosenthal, R. and R. Rosnow (eds.)
1970    *Sources of Artifact in Social Research.* New York: Academic Press.

Rueschemeyer, D.
1964    "Doctors and lawyers: a comment on the theory of the professions." *Canadian Review of Sociology and Anthropology* 1:17–30.

Schatzman, L. and A.L. Strauss
1973    *Field Research: Strategies for a Natural Sociology.* Englewood Cliffs, N.J.: Prentice-Hall.

Schanck, R.L.
1932    "A study of a community and its groups and institutions conceived of as behaviors of individuals." *Psychological Monographs* 43, 2.

Scott, M.B.
1968    *The Racing Game.* Chicago: Aldine.

Shaffir, W., V. Marshall and J. Haas
1980    "Competing commitments: unanticipated problems of field research." *Qualitative Sociology,* 2:56–71.

Shibutani, T.
1966    *Improvised News: A Sociological Study of Rumor.* Indianapolis: Bobbs-Merrill.

Shipman, M. (ed.)
1976    *The Organization and Impact of Social Research.* London: Routledge & Kegan Paul.
Siegler, M. and H. Osmond
1973    "Aesculapian authority." *Hastings Center Studies* 1:41–52.
Simmel, G.
1950    "The triad." Pp. in K.H. Wolff (ed.) *The Sociology of Georg Simmel.* New York: Free Press.
Simpson, M.
1972    *Medical Education: A Critical Approach.* London: Butterworth.
Spaulding, W.B.
1969    "The undergraduate medical curriculum (1969 model): McMaster University." *Canadian Medical Association Journal* 100:659–664.
Strauss, A.L., L. Schatzman, R. Bucher, D. Ehrlich, and M. Sabshin
1964    *Psychiatric Ideologies and Institutions.* New York: Free Press.
Sweeney, G.D. and D.L. Mitchell
1975    "An introduction to the study of medicine: phase 1 of the McMaster M.D. program." *Journal of Medical Education* 50: 70–77.
Turner, V.
1970    *The Ritual Process: Structure and Anti-Structure.* Chicago: Aldine.
Valentine, C.
1968    *Culture and Poverty.* Chicago: University of Chicago Press.
Vidich, A.J., J. Bensman, and M.R. Stein (eds.)
1964    *Reflections on Community Studies.* New York: Harper & Row.
Walsh, W.J.
1978    "The McMaster programme of medical education, Hamilton, Ontario, Canada: developing problem-solving abilities." Pp. 69–79 in F.M. Katz and T. Fülöp (eds.) *Personnel for Health Care: Case Studies of Educational Programmes.* Public Health Papers, 70, World Health Organization, Geneva.
Watson, J.D.
1969    *The Double Helix: A Personal Account of the Discovery of the D.N.A., by James D. Watson.* New York: New American Library.
Whyte, W.F.
1955    *Street Corner Society.* Chicago: University of Chicago Press.
Wilensky, H.R.
1964    "The professionalization of everyone?" *American Journal of Sociology* 70 (2): 137–158.
Yancy, W.L. and L. Rainwater
1970    "Problems in the ethnography of the urban under-class." Pp.245–269 in R. Habenstein (ed.) *Pathways to Data: Field Methods for Studying On-going Social Organizations.* Chicago: Aldine.
Zimmerman, D.H. and D.L. Wieder
1977    "The diary: diary-interview method." *Urban Life* 5:479–498.

# Index